369 0246752

This book is due for return on or before the last date shown below.

NEUROLOGIC OUTCOMES OF SURGERY AND ANESTHESIA

NEUROLOGIC OUTCOMES
OF SURGERY AND
ANESTHESIA

EDITED BY

George A. Mashour, MD, PhD

ASSOCIATE CHAIR FOR FACULTY AFFAIRS

ASSOCIATE PROFESSOR OF ANESTHESIOLOGY

AND NEUROSURGERY

FACULTY, NEUROSCIENCE GRADUATE PROGRAM

UNIVERSITY OF MICHIGAN MEDICAL SCHOOL

ANN ARBOR, MICHIGAN

EDITED BY

Michael S. Avidan, MB BCh,
FCASA

PROFESSOR OF ANESTHESIOLOGY AND SURGERY

DIRECTOR, INSTITUTE OF QUALITY IMPROVEMENT,

RESEARCH & INFORMATICS

DIVISION CHIEF, CARDIOTHORACIC ANESTHESIOLOGY

WASHINGTON UNIVERSITY SCHOOL OF MEDICINE

ST. LOUIS, MISSOURI

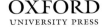

OXFORD
UNIVERSITY PRESS

Oxford University Press is a department of the University of Oxford.
It furthers the University's objective of excellence in research, scholarship,
and education by publishing worldwide.

Oxford   New York
Auckland   Cape Town   Dar es Salaam   Hong Kong   Karachi
Kuala Lumpur   Madrid   Melbourne   Mexico City   Nairobi
New Delhi   Shanghai   Taipei   Toronto

With offices in
Argentina   Austria   Brazil   Chile   Czech Republic   France   Greece
Guatemala   Hungary   Italy   Japan   Poland   Portugal   Singapore
South Korea   Switzerland   Thailand   Turkey   Ukraine   Vietnam

Oxford is a registered trademark of Oxford University Press in the UK and certain other
countries.

Published in the United States of America by
Oxford University Press
198 Madison Avenue, New York, NY 10016

Library of Congress Cataloging-in-Publication Data
Neurologic outcomes of surgery and anesthesia/edited by George A. Mashour, Michael S. Avidan.
    p. ; cm.
Includes bibliographical references and index.
ISBN 978-0-19-989572-4—ISBN 978-0-19-998593-7—ISBN 978-0-19-998594-4
I. Mashour, George A. (George Alexander), 1969–   II. Avidan, Michael.
[DNLM: 1. Nervous System Diseases—etiology.   2. Anesthesia—adverse effects.   3. Postoperative Complications. WL 140]
617.9′6748—dc23   2012036330

This material is not intended to be, and should not be considered, a substitute for medical or other professional advice. Treatment for the conditions described in this material is highly dependent on the individual circumstances. And, while this material is designed to offer accurate information with respect to the subject matter covered and to be current as of the time it was written, research and knowledge about medical and health issues is constantly evolving and dose schedules for medications are being revised continually, with new side effects recognized and accounted for regularly. Readers must therefore always check the product information and clinical procedures with the most up-to-date published product information and data sheets provided by the manufacturers and the most recent codes of conduct and safety regulation. The publisher and the authors make no representations or warranties to readers, express or implied, as to the accuracy or completeness of this material. Without limiting the foregoing, the publisher and the authors make no representations or warranties as to the accuracy or efficacy of the drug dosages mentioned in the material. The authors and the publisher do not accept, and expressly disclaim, any responsibility for any liability, loss or risk that may be claimed or incurred as a consequence of the use and/or application of any of the contents of this material.

9 8 7 6 5 4 3 2 1
Printed in China on acid-free paper

*Dedicated to our fathers, Alexander Mashour (1929–2010) and
Jos Avidan (1929–2012)—two free spirits who played by their own rules*

CONTENTS

PREFACE

The latter half of the twentieth century saw a dramatic improvement in perioperative outcomes, in large part because of the development of safer drugs and the standardization of intraoperative monitoring. It is striking, however, that the standard monitors in current use are limited to the cardiovascular and respiratory systems, when it is the nervous system that is the primary target of the therapeutic effects of general anesthesia. Indeed, during the twentieth century attention was focused on the cardiopulmonary outcomes of surgery, with significantly less attention paid to the brain and other neural structures. The consequent improvement in cardiopulmonary outcomes led to a new standard of safety and a new horizon of outcomes research.

The perioperative physicians and investigators of the twenty-first century are now recognizing the need for more extensive study of neurologic outcomes. However, this endeavor is proving to be a significant challenge, for several reasons. First, there are no standard intraoperative monitors for the brain or nervous system. Thus, unlike the electrocardiogram, which can detect intraoperative *myocardial* ischemia, we do not routinely use an electroencephalogram or other brain monitor that might detect intraoperative *cerebral* ischemia. Second, there is a notable lack of biomarkers for the nervous system, which limits the large-scale study of neurologic outcomes. There are a number of commonly assessed quantitative markers for heart or kidney damage, but there is nothing comparable to troponin or creatinine for the brain or spinal cord. Furthermore, some outcomes relate to subtle functional abilities that may not even be reflected in abnormal neural biomarker levels. More subtle deficits in cognition, for example, require careful, costly, and labor-intensive examinations by trained professionals, creating obstacles for large-scale studies. The third challenge is that the nervous system is not functionally homogenous. Unlike the heart that serves primarily as a pump, the nervous system (even the brain itself) has tremendous functional specialization, rendering it almost impossible to treat it as

a single organ for the purposes of outcomes studies. Finally, there are still a number of fundamental mysteries regarding neural function. Indeed, one reason we do not have a standard monitor for the brain is that there is an incomplete understanding of what is best to measure and where.

Despite the challenges—or, rather, because of them—neurologic and psychiatric outcomes of surgery, as well as the potentially neurotoxic effects of general anesthetics, are a subject of intense and often controversial inquiry. Where can the interested clinician or investigator turn for a concise introduction to the issues at hand? *Neurologic Outcomes of Surgery and Anesthesia* provides, for the first time, a concise and clear resource for information on virtually all major neurologic and psychiatric outcomes, including delirium, stroke, posttraumatic stress disorder, spinal cord injury, postoperative visual loss, and more. Furthermore, general topics of interest such as neurotoxicity, neuromonitoring, and neurologic biomarkers are addressed. Internationally recognized experts who have made important contributions to the primary literature of the field have been selected to write high-yield chapters in a standardized format that enhances clarity. We thank these scholars and clinicians for their outstanding work, which we believe has resulted in a cutting-edge and readable textbook that will bring together in a single volume the many neurologic complications of surgery and anesthesia that previously were treated as individual topics.

The brain in particular—and the nervous system in general—is often regarded as the final frontier of the biological sciences because of its complexity, functional heterogeneity, and sensitivity to injury. Similarly, we feel that the nervous system is the final frontier of perioperative medicine and hope that *Neurologic Outcomes of Surgery and Anesthesia* creates new awareness of this exciting field as well as a renewed sense of importance in protecting the nervous system from injury during surgery and beyond.

— George A. Mashour and Michael S. Avidan

CONTRIBUTORS

Rae M. Allain, MD
Associate Director, Surgical Critical Care
Department of Anesthesiology and
    Pain Medicine
St. Elizabeth's Medical Center
Boston, Massachusetts

Michael S. Avidan, MB BCh, FCASA
Professor of Anesthesiology and Surgery
Director, Institute of Quality Improvement, Research &
    Informatics
Division Chief, Cardiothoracic Anesthesiology
Washington University School of Medicine
St. Louis, Missouri

Ansgar M. Brambrink MD, PhD
Professor, Department of Anesthesiology & Perioperative
    Medicine
Oregon Health & Science University
Portland, Oregon

Gary J. Brenner, MD, PhD
Director of the MGH Pain Medicine
    Fellowship
Massachusetts General Hospital
Department of Anesthesia, Critical Care and Pain
    Medicine; and
Assistant Professor in Anesthesia
Harvard Medical School
Boston, Massachusetts

Chad M. Brummett, MD
Assistant Professor
Director, Pain Research
Department of Anesthesiology
Division of Pain Medicine
University of Michigan
Ann Arbor, Michigan

Juan P. Cata, MD
Assistant Professor, Department of Anesthesiology and
    Perioperative Medicine
Section of Neuroanesthesia
University of Texas
MD Anderson Cancer Center
Houston, Texas

Alex S. Evers, MD
Henry E. Mallinckrodt Professor, Anesthesiology
Head, Department of Anesthesiology
Washington University School of Medicine
St. Louis, Missouri

Robert S. Griffin, MD, PhD
Department of Anesthesiology
Division of Musculoskeletal and Interventional Pain
    Management
Hospital For Special Surgery
New York, New York

Sharon K. Inouye, MD, MPH
Professor, Department of Medicine
Harvard Medical School; and
Director, Aging Brain Center
Institute for Aging Research
Hebrew SeniorLife
Boston, Massachusetts

Adam K. Jacob, MD
Assistant Professor, Department of Anesthesiology
Mayo Clinic
Rochester, Minnesota

Elliott Karren, MD
Department of Anesthesiology
Washington University School of Medicine
St. Louis, Missouri

Antoun Koht, MD
Professor of Anesthesiology, Neurological Surgery and
    Neurology
Northwestern University Medical School
Chicago, Illinois

Sandra L. Kopp, MD
Associate Professor, Department of Anesthesiology
Mayo Clinic
Rochester, Minnesota

Lorri A. Lee, MD
Professor, Departments of Anesthesiology and Pain
    Medicine, and Neurologic Surgery (adjunct)
University of Washington
Seattle, Washington

Mazen A. Maktabi, MD
Chief, Division of General Surgery Anesthesia
Department of Anesthesia, Critical Care, and Pain
    Medicine
Massachusetts General Hospital
Harvard Medical School
Boston, Massachusetts

George A. Mashour, MD, PhD
Associate Chair for Faculty Affairs
Associate Professor of Anesthesiology and Neurosurgery
Faculty, Neuroscience Graduate Program
University of Michigan Medical School
Ann Arbor, Michigan

Mervyn Maze, MD
Professor and Chair, Department of Anesthesia and
    Perioperative Care
University of California, San Francisco
San Francisco, California

Laurel E. Moore, MD
Clinical Assistant Professor, Department of
    Anesthesiology
Assistant Clinical Director, University Hospital Operating
    Rooms
Director, Neuroanesthesiology
University of Michigan Medical School
Ann Arbor, Michigan

Lewis B. Morgenstern, MD
Professor, Neurology
University of Michigan Medical School
Ann Arbor, Michigan

Adam D. Niesen, MD
Assistant Professor, Department of Anesthesiology
Mayo Clinic
Rochester, Minnesota

Vijay Kumar Rimaiah, MBBS, MD
Acting Instructor and Senior Fellow, Department of
    Anesthesiology and Pain Medicine
University of Washington
Seattle, Washington

Thomas L. Rodebaugh, PhD
Assistant Professor, Department of Psychology
Washington University School of Medicine
St. Louis, Missouri

Robert Sanders, MD
Senior Clinical Research Associate, Imaging
    Neuroscience
Institute of Neurology
Faculty of Brain Sciences
University College London
London, England

Rehan Siddiqui, MD
Department of Anesthesia, Critical Care, and Pain
    Medicine
Massachusetts General Hospital
Harvard Medical School
Boston, Massachusetts

Tod B. Sloan, MD, MBA, PhD
Professor of Anesthesiology
University of Colorado School of Medicine
Aurora, Colorado

J. Richard Toleikis, PhD
Associate Professor of Anesthesiology
Rush University Medical School
Chicago, Illinois

Marnie B. Welch, MD
Department of Anesthesiology
Dartmouth Hitchcock Medical Center
Lebanon, New Hampshire

Elizabeth L. Whitlock, MD, MSc
Department of Anesthesia and Perioperative Care
University of California
San Francisco Medical Center
San Francisco, California

PART I

BRAIN

1.

ANESTHETIC NEUROTOXICITY

EFFECTS OF ANESTHETIC DRUGS ON THE DEVELOPING BRAIN

Ansgar M. Brambrink

INTRODUCTION TO THE CLINICAL PROBLEM

While over many decades the field of anesthesiology has developed safe strategies to provide anesthesia to infants and children, thereby radically improving perioperative care and surgical outcomes in the young, there currently is growing concern that most of today's typically used anesthetics might be harmful to the developing brain. Evidence is mounting that exposure to sedative and anesthetic agents injures brain cells and could potentially cause persistent neurocognitive deficits that present as inappropriate behaviors, leaning difficulties, and specific neuropsychological syndromes.[1]

Pediatric anesthesiologists and intensive care clinicians face a difficult dilemma. On the one hand, strong evidence from the laboratory promotes the view that many sedatives and anesthetics are harmful to the developing brain of several species, including nonhuman primates.[2,3] In contrast, comparable data pertaining to humans are not available, and the clinical evidence is ambiguous and currently based on retrospective epidemiologic studies.[4] The conundrum for health care providers and patients is that virtually all currently available anesthetic agents appear to cause harm in animal models, and there are no proven safe alternatives on the horizon.

It is now accepted that infants and neonates experience pain and stress. Providing them adequate analgesia and sedation during surgery reduces the risk that they will acquire hyperalgesia,[5] developmental brain alterations,[6] and inappropriate behaviors.[7–9] Nevertheless, prolonged exposure to some of the very agents that are available to treat pain, provide sedation, and maintain anesthesia may be harmful to human fetuses and infants. Such exposure could potentially produce the outcomes that occur following the experience of pain and stress without alleviating medication. This paradox is stimulating discussions regarding the risk-to-benefit relationship of providing human neonates and young infants with anesthetic and sedative medications for painful or stressful procedures.[10] The relevance of anesthetic-induced neurotoxicity to developing humans is currently unclear; therefore, to date no practice changes have been advocated. However, both in society and among health care practitioners, awareness is growing about the potential neurotoxicity of anesthetic agents to developing humans. It is essential that the clinical relevance of anesthetic neurotoxicity be clarified and that the safety of specific sedative, analgesic, and anesthetic drugs be explored. Two prospective clinical studies are under way, which aim to answer some of the burning questions related to this issue[11,12] (for review, see Stratmann [2011][3]), such as whether regional anesthesia is safer than general anesthesia. Consortiums between government and scientific organizations have been created to guide the discussions between professionals and society, as well as to support research and development aimed at resolving this perceived public health problem as expeditiously as possible[13,14] (for more detailed information see http://www.smarttots.org).

INCIDENCE, PREVALENCE, AND OUTCOMES

Since the first descriptions of toxic effects of neuroactive drugs in the developing brain,[15–17] strong evidence has been provided by multiple studies that anesthetic drugs currently used in humans cause widespread neuroapoptosis in immature mice, rats, pigs, guinea pigs, and nonhuman primates.[15–36] This injury occurs in developing animal brains at doses and durations that are clinically relevant and is associated with long-term neurocognitive deficits weeks to months after the exposure.

While initially challenged regarding validity and relevance,[37–39] the evidence from animal studies pointing toward a significant problem has gained acceptance, first because several independent groups have reproduced the findings of neuroapoptosis, and second as evidence is consistent across mammalian species, including nonhuman primates. Nevertheless, it remains a matter of discussion whether the animal findings are relevant to the human situation, and it will take several years before results from these prospective clinical trials are available.

The best available human evidence comes from epidemiologic studies. While the data are inconclusive, several retrospective analyses suggest that anesthesia exposure during infancy may increase risk for neurobehavioral disturbances. Emerging evidence suggests that age at exposure, number of exposures, and total duration of anesthesia may all be associated with worse neurobehavioral outcomes.

DiMaggio and co-workers at Columbia University analyzed data of children enrolled in Medicaid in order to identify those who were exposed to brief general anesthesia before 3 years of age. Their results demonstrate that exposure to anesthesia more than doubles the risk of being diagnosed with behavioral disorders during later development compared to matched children who were not exposed. Moreover, the risk was even higher in children exposed twice or more during the first 3 years of life.[40] Analysis of a birth cohort of siblings nested in the this study suggested that the risk of being diagnosed with developmental and behavioral disorders was 60% greater than that of a similar group of siblings who did not undergo surgery before 3 years of life.[41]

Wilder, Flick, and co-workers at the Mayo Clinic evaluated county-based data for children who had received anesthesia prior to 4 years of age. Their analysis indicated no measurable risk for learning disabilities when young children received a single general anesthetic. In contrast, children anesthetized twice or more were at increased risk for learning disabilities. Additionally, anesthesia duration of longer than 120 minutes was associated with the highest risk.[42] Adjustment for comorbidity confirmed these results and suggested a two-fold higher hazard ratio for developing a learning disability with two or more anesthesia exposures (median duration 75 minutes) before the age of 2 years.[43] Most recently, the same group using the same data sources showed that repeated exposure to general anesthesia before age 2 years more than doubles the risk for the diagnosis of attention-deficit/hyperactivity disorder until age 19 years, even after adjusting for comorbidities.[44]

Thomas and co-workers from the University of Iowa reported data from a smaller sample that produced results along the same line. Brief anesthesia before 1 year of age doubled the risk of scoring below the 5th percentile in school achievement tests compared to the population norm. Moreover, the poorest academic performance was observed in those children exposed to the longest duration of anesthesia.[45]

Kalkman and co-workers from the University of Utrecht in The Netherlands also reported a higher incidence of subsequent neurocognitive impairments when anesthesia was provided to infants than that among children older than 1 year at the time of exposure.[46]

Hansen and co-workers from the Odense University in Denmark reported from a large cohort of Danish adolescents that there was no evidence of impaired academic achievement in those who had undergone one brief anesthetic (30–60 minutes) at 1 year of age or younger.[47]

Bartels and co-workers from the Vrije University in Amsterdam analyzed data from The Netherlands Twin Registry and found that monozygotic twins who were exposed to anesthesia before age 3, according to parental report, had significantly lower educational achievement scores and significantly more cognitive problems than twins not exposed to anesthesia. However, in those twin pairs in which one twin was exposed to anesthesia and the other twin was not, the academic achievements were similar between the two.[48]

It is remarkable that several large and reasonably well-controlled, yet still retrospective, studies document an association between brief exposure to anesthesia in early life and neurobehavioral disturbances later in life. While these studies certainly prove relevance for further investigation in humans, at this point it is not possible to prove a causal relationship based on theses retrospective studies because of their inherent methodologic limitations and their limited focus.

For instance, all of these studies are based on secondary analyses of observational data that had been collected usually for other purposes, and some include information from parental interviews. Another concern is that all data sources describe anesthesia-relevant information that dates back several decades (1970–1980s). Since then, anesthesia practice has changed significantly. For example, the volatile anesthetic agent halothane is rarely used today in developed countries, and monitoring devices that were unavailable 30 years ago are standard care today (e.g., quantitative measurements of anesthetic gases; capnometry and capnography; peripheral oxygen saturation measurement via pulse oximetry). The focus of several investigations was limited to subjects exposed only briefly to anesthetic drugs. While their population-based approach removes certain biases, none of them provides information about the indication for anesthesia and the drugs used, and some provide no information about the number of exposures, the duration of exposure, or whether investigators attempted to control for confounders such as socioeconomic status or family conditions. Prolonged durations of exposure, combinations of different drugs, and developmental age at exposure are all likely important determinants of severity and pattern of neuropathologic and neurobehavioral outcome after early anesthesia exposure, but these factors require more detailed evaluation. Two large, prospective human trials are under way, and their results might help clarify some of the risk factors for bad outcomes and answer whether and to what extent early exposure to general anesthesia might cause long-term adverse neurobehavioral sequelae.[49–52]

RISK FACTORS

Key risk factors are the type of drugs and the drug combinations to which the developing brain is exposed. Anesthesia-induced developmental neuroapoptosis was first observed after exposure of infant rodents to drugs that block the N-methyl-D-aspartate (NMDA) subtype of glutamate receptors.[15] Subsequent research in the same model showed an even more pronounced apoptogenic potency for ethanol, which both blocks NMDA receptors and promotes neurotransmission at γ-aminobutyric acid (GABA$_A$) receptors.[16] Research was quickly extended to include other drugs that interact with GABA$_A$ and NMDA receptors as agonist and antagonist, respectively, known targets for many anesthetics and sedatives. Studies showed similar deleterious effects when clinically relevant doses of ketamine,[17] midazolam,[17] propofol,[23] isoflurane,[22,26,27] sevoflurane,[24,25] desflurane,[27,53] and chloral hydrate,[54] as well as antiepileptic drugs, including those that block voltage-gated sodium channels,[55] were administered to infant rodents. Moreover, combinations of NMDA antagonists with GABA$_A$-mimetic drugs potentiated the neuroapoptotic effects.[17,19,20]

Recent evidence suggests that some nonanesthetic/ nonsedatives that are used clinically, such as caffeine, may be able to augment the deleterious effects of NMDA antagonists and GABA$_A$-mimetic drugs. Caffeine, a nonselective adenosine receptor antagonist and an inhibitor of acetylcholine esterase, increased apoptotic cell death associated with exposure to alcohol,[56] anesthetics like isoflurane,[57,58] and sedatives like benzodiazipines[59] in several experimental models. The clinical relevance of these findings is that some preterm infants are treated for weeks with caffeine to stimulate their respiratory drive in the intensive care environment to treat apnea.[60] At the same time many of these infants also receive sedatives to relieve distress or anesthetics to induce tolerance for necessary procedures. Still other preterm infants are treated short term in the context of general anesthesia in order to reduce the risk for postoperative apnea.

A probable key risk factor for neurotoxic effects of anesthetics is age at exposure. Evidence from the laboratory suggests that the period of peak vulnerability coincides with the "brain growth spurt," which varies between species and is characterized by rapid synaptogenesis.[15,16] In rodents this developmental period is considered to occur in the early postnatal period. In contrast, in humans synaptogenesis continues from about mid-gestation to several years after birth,[61,62] thus vulnerability to anesthetics in humans could extend long beyond infancy. Retrospective studies in humans suggest an increased risk for neurobehavioral deficits when anesthesia is provided to patients under the age of 1–4 years. Studies in nonhuman primates support the concerns about an extended period of vulnerability. Ketamine anesthesia in the pregnant rhesus monkey at the beginning of the third trimester induced fetal neuroapoptosis.[29,35] Anesthesia with isoflurane,[31,32,36] ketamine,[30,32,35] or nitrous oxide plus isoflurane[33] resulted in apoptotic cell death in 5- to 6-day-old rhesus macaques.

When comparing neurodevelopmental milestones, a third-trimester rhesus fetus corresponds approximately to a human neonate. A 5- to 6-day-old rhesus infant is approximately equivalent to a 6-month old human infant.[62,63] It is unclear whether the window of vulnerability indeed closes at that time or is species dependent and for certain subgroups of brain cells remains open for a significantly longer period of brain development.

Another issue that has not been systematically studied is whether the developing brain has a differential sensitivity to the apoptogenic action of anesthetic drugs during the fetal and neonatal periods. Our own preliminary findings in nonhuman primates indicate that isoflurane induces more severe damage in the neonatal brain than in the fetal brain. In contrast, ketamine is more toxic for the fetal brain than for the neonatal brain. These observations underscore the interdependence of both the developmental age at the time of exposure and the class of anesthetic drug administered. Evidence that ketamine (and perhaps other NMDA antagonists, including alcohol[64]) may be more toxic when exposure occurs prenatally suggests that we need to focus future human studies on in utero fetuses and premature infants.

A precise delineation of the peak vulnerability also requires an understanding of the key mechanisms that lead to persistent neurobehavioral deficits at a later age. While several studies in rodents[17,18,20,25,65–67] and one "proof-of-concept" study in nonhuman primates[34] document that exposure to anesthesia early in life has long-term neurocognitive consequences, it remains unknown whether the functional deficits result from injury to neurons, to glia, or to the proliferating stem cell pool, or whether an impaired ability to create cell-to-cell contact is responsible.

Neuroapoptosis has been shown to result from exposure to different anesthetics as well as to alcohol during fetal and neonatal life in rodents and in other species, including guinea pig,[28] piglet,[68] and nonhuman primate.[29–36,64] No brain region is completely spared, but the brain regions sustaining the most severe neuronal losses are regions that receive and integrate sensory information through both visual and auditory association pathways, which are critically important for normal neurocognitive function. Our own data showed that thalamus and basal ganglia were severely damaged in fetal brain of nonhuman primates exposed to anesthetics in utero. This closely mirrors findings in human children[69–71] who were exposed in utero to alcohol or antiepileptic drugs, both of which are neurotoxic to the developing brain. Anesthetic exposure appears to affect particularly glutamatergic, GABAergic, and dopaminergic neurons in the developing brain but spares cholinergic neurons in the basal forebrain.[72]

Glia cells also have been found to be sensitive, as evidenced from recent observations of robust apoptosis involving young oligodendroglia following exposure to alcohol[73] or anesthetic drugs[32,36] in the developing brain of rodent and nonhuman primates. Deletion of young oligodendrocytes that are just beginning to myelinate axons, which interconnect neurons throughout the developing brain, could potentially have adverse long-term neurobehavioral consequences, which might be additive to those of anesthesia-induced neuroapoptosis.[36] It also remains unclear whether the window of oligodendroglial vulnerability to anesthetic exposure parallels that of neurons or is further extended, given the ongoing myelination in later childhood.

Exposure to anesthetics apparently also affects neuronal dendrites and synapsis. Isoflurane has been shown to reduce the number of immature dendritic spines in vitro and the number of synapses in vivo of infant mice, which is likely mediated by isoflurane-induced p75 receptor signaling.[74,75] Furthermore, Briner and co-workers showed that isoflurane, sevoflurane, desflurane, and propofol all reduce synaptic spine density in newborn rodents; but when given to older infant rodents (16–25 days old), the same drugs actually increased spine density and synaptogenesis.[76–78]

Proliferation and differentiation of new neurons appear sensitive to anesthetics in an age-dependent fashion. Rodents exposed at a young age showed a persistent impairment of neurogenesis that was associated with neurocognitive deficits later in life.[79,80] In particular, multiple brief isoflurane exposures to rats and mice on postnatal days 14–17 caused a reduction in dentate hippocampal neurons and neurocognitive impairment that became progressively more severe with advancing age.[80] Other investigators have provided evidence that neonatal exposure of rodents to ethanol[81] or to various sedatives and anticonvulsants[82] suppresses neurogenesis in the dentate hippocampal gyrus, which is associated with a permanent reduction in the number of dentate hippocampal neurons and with persistent neurocognitive deficits as the animals mature. Interestingly, the vulnerability for anesthesia-induced impairment of neurogenesis appears to extend past the second postnatal week in mice[80] and thereby lasts longer than the window of vulnerability currently assumed for anesthesia-induced neuroapoptosis.

It seems likely that each of these injury mechanisms has a specific period of peak vulnerability; further research is needed to provide more evidence.

PREVENTIVE STRATEGIES AND TREATMENT

Researchers have identified several compounds and strategies that limit the extent of anesthesia-induced neuroapoptosis in vitro and in vivo experimental models. However, no evidence is available from clinical studies.

It is accepted by many that the anesthesia-induced cell death morphologically and in terms of temporal manifestation is consistent with programmed cell death (apoptosis) and involves mechanisms shown as characteristic for apoptotic cell death induced by other injury mechanisms.[15–17,83–85] In vitro and in vivo studies have demonstrated that exposure to anesthetics is associated with a reduction of elements involved in prosurvival signaling cascades such as phosphorylated extracellular signal-regulated protein kinase (pERK),[86–88] Bclx[L],[88,89] and Bcl-2.[90–93] It is also associated with upregulation of cell death–promoting signaling involving Bax,[94] p53[93] protein expression, increased levels of hypoxia-inducible factor-1a protein,[95] as well as mitochondrial injury and extramitochondrial leakage of cytochrome c.[89–94] This is followed by a sequence of intracellular changes culminating in activation of caspase-3[19,94,96,97] and also may involve neurotrophic factor (BDNF)-dependent[94,96,98] and death receptor-dependent pathways[99,100] leading to cell destruction. Others have proposed that anesthetic-induced neuronal injury, at least in rat brains, is the result of an excitotoxic mechanism.[101] This line of evidence suggests that, based on differences in cellular chloride gradients secondary to the ontogenetic timing of ion-transporter protein expression, GABA$_A$ receptor activation in the immature rat brain essentially results in excitation of the neuronal circuitry until a shift to a hyperpolarizing action of GABA$_A$ receptor activation occurs after about the second postnatal week.[102–104]

On the basis of the models mentioned above, several neuroprotective strategies have been experimentally tested, including single-dose treatment with lithium (blocks the reduction of pERK concentration[87]) or melantonin (mitochondria membrane stabilizer[89]); the coadministration of xenon (increases Bcl-2 and reduces cytochrome C release and p53 activation[90,93]), dexmedetomidine (reverses Bcl-2 and pERK reduction[91,92]), or L-carnitine (an antioxidant[105]); the experimental blockade of neuronal chloride uptake, the driving force for depolarizing GABA$_A$ receptor–mediated responses in immature neurons, via inhibition of Na-K-2Cl cotransporter 1 using bumetanide,[106] or interference with the deleterious signaling of uncleaved proBDNF at the p75 neurotrophin receptor using specific inhibitors (Pep5 or Fc-p75[74,75]).

However, for most of these interventions, it remains unknown whether they also ameliorate the subsequent neurobehavioral effects of anesthesia exposure at young age. In fact, bumetanide treatment did not alleviate sevoflurane-induced functional impairment (in vitro electrophysiological recordings of long-term potentiation on day 14–17 after exposure) while it protected against the early sevoflurane-induced caspase-3 activation.[106] In contrast, Sanders and co-workers reported that dexmedetomidine coadministration reduced isoflurane-induced neuronal apoptosis (caspase-3 activation) and also completely prevented the memory impairment that was apparent in the 40-day-old rats, which were exposed to isoflurane alone on postnatal day 7.[91] Others have reported beneficial effects of recombinant erythropoietin, which was coadministered during anesthesia, and ameliorated isoflurane-induced neurodegeneration as well as the learning deficits in infant mice.[107]

Recently, the application of anesthetics under hypothermic conditions was evaluated in pilot experiments that document a complete suppression of neuroapoptosis following isoflurane and ketamine exposure.[108] Hypothermia is becoming more accepted as a therapeutic means to improve outcome after cardiac arrest and hypoxic-ischemic injury in neonates, which is based on its ability to reduce immediate cell death in acute substrate deprivation. In contrast, cell death induced by anesthetics is strictly apoptotic and requires the execution of specific cellular programs, which may be suppressed during hypothermia.

Thus, it is critical that future research determine whether hypothermia protects permanently against anesthesia-induced cell injury or just postpones the initiation of the process.

Most recently, Shih and co-workers suggested that anesthesia-induced cognitive decline in rats could be treated with adequate sensory and cognitive stimulation, including voluntary exercise.[67] They based their conclusions on observations that animals exposed to 4 hours of sevoflurane on postnatal day 7 and released into an enriched environment starting 4 weeks after anesthesia had improved cognitive function at 8 weeks postanesthesia compared to those animals that remained in the deprived standard laboratory environment. Interestingly, the neurocognitive capacity of control animals that spent the 4 weeks in the enriched environment also improved, and at 8 weeks both the anesthesia-exposed animals and the control animals performed similarly.[67] Future research is required to determine the relevance of these findings, the targeted injury, and the potential therapeutic intervention, since human children at baseline are exposed to an incredibly enriched environment compared to that of rodents in the laboratory.

CURRENT GUIDELINES AND RECOMMENDATIONS

Currently, mounting experimental evidence suggests that sedatives and anesthetics have toxic effects on the developing brain, causing long-term neurobehavioral impairment and permanent neuropathologic changes in animals exposed to these drugs in the first weeks of their life.

For humans, retrospective data analysis points to an association between exposure to anesthesia at a young age (<3 years of age) and neurobehavioral disturbances during later development, but the same data do not allow us to determine whether this is a causal relationship. Thus, today's evidence is not strong enough to suggest any guidelines or recommendations for the practice of anesthesiology.

Moreover, it remains entirely unknown whether certain drugs among those currently available to provide sedation and anesthesia are safer than others. Such comparisons have not been made in humans, and no database exists to allow a retrospective analysis. Given the current uncertainty regarding the relevance of the experimental findings for the human condition, it seems premature to pursue clinical research that aims to identify safe versus less safe practice of anesthesia.

First, well-designed and executed clinical studies are needed to determine whether brains of human children are at risk for toxic effects of anesthetics and to determine the neurocognitive consequences of such an exposure. On the basis of those results, comparative clinical research could identify safe practice for pediatric anesthesia, and the direction of such research could be informed by data from experimental research, particular in nonhuman primates. It is highly likely that the results will suggest an age-specific approach, identify acceptable exposure times, drug combinations, and protective means and reliable postexposure biomarker screening technology (for an example of emerging concepts see Makaryus et al.[109]). It is also quite likely that new anesthetics and sedatives will emerge that will be proven safer than those used today.

Once these milestones have been reached, enough evidence will be available to create recommendations and guidelines that could change current clinical practice.

CONCLUSION

Evidence for anesthetic neurotoxicity in the developing brain of a variety of different mammal species, including nonhuman primates, has accumulated to the point that the existence of the phenomenon is indisputable. However, knowledge about the underlying mechanisms is still scarce, and the discussion continues as to whether human infants and children are at risk for anesthetic neurotoxicity.[110–112] Currently, there is no evidence from clinical research that could guide a change in clinical practice, and results from experimental studies require clinical verification before change could be advocated for safety. Moreover, even if clinical evidence were available to fundamentally challenge current perioperative practice for parturients, infants, and children and to demonstrate that anesthetics render dose-dependent neurotoxic effects on the developing brain, the lack of alternatives to the current practice poses a considerable challenge to the health care system as a whole. Changes in drug selection, dosage, and duration might then be considered if no pharmacologic tools were available to allow for the provision of anesthesia without neurotoxic effects to the young brain.

Meanwhile, it is imperative to conduct well-designed human trials to determine the clinical risk as well as the key confounding variables. It is also important to support highly relevant translational research that focuses on prevention of anesthetic neurotoxicity, on noninvasive diagnosis of injury, on postexposure treatment, and on pharmacologic innovation in order to successfully tackle this critical problem.

CONFLICT OF INTEREST STATEMENT

"A.B. has no conflicts of interest to disclose."

REFERENCES

1. Kuehn BM. FDA considers data on potential risks of anesthesia use in infants, children. *JAMA*. 2011;305(17):1749–1750, 1753.
2. Hughes CG, Pandharipande PP. The effects of perioperative and intensive care unit sedation on brain organ dysfunction [review]. *Anesth Analg*. 2011;112(5):1212–1217.
3. Stratmann G. Neurotoxicity of anesthetic drugs in the developing brain [review]. *Anesth Analg*. 2011;113:1170–1179.
4. Sun L. Early childhood general anaesthesia exposure and neurocognitive development. *Br J Anaesth*. 2010;105(Suppl 1):i61–i68.
5. Ruda MA, Ling QD, Hohmann AG, Peng YB, Tachibana T. Altered nociceptive neuronal circuits after neonatal peripheral inflammation. *Science*. 2000;289: 628–631.
6. Anand KJ, Scalzo FM Can adverse neonatal experiences alter brain development and subsequent behavior? *Biol Neonate*. 2000;77:69–82.
7. Simons SH, van Dijk M, Anand KJS, Roofthooft D, van Lingen RA, Tibboell D. Do we still hurt newborn babies? A prospective study of procedural pain and analgesia in neonates. *Arch Pediatr Adolesc Med*. 2003;157:1058–1064.
8. Bouza H. The impact of pain in the immature brain. *J Matern Fetal Neonatal Med*. 2009;22:722–732.
9. Huang W, Deprest J, Missant C, Van de Velde M. Management of fetal pain during invasive fetal procedures: a review. *Acta Anaesthesiol Belg*. 2004;55:119–123.
10. Davidson AJ. Neurotoxicity and the need for anesthesia in the newborn: does the emperor have no clothes? *Anesthesiology*. 2012;116(3):507–509.
11. Davidson AJ, McCann ME, Morton NS, Myles PS. Anesthesia and outcome after neonatal surgery: the role for randomized trials. *Anesthesiology*. 2008;109:941–944.
12. Sun LS, Li G, Dimaggio C, et al. Anesthesia and neurodevelopment in children: time for an answer? *Anesthesiology*. 2008;109:757–761.
13. Jevtovic-Todorovic V. Pediatric anesthesia neurotoxicity: an overview of the 2011 SmartTots panel. *Anesth Analg*. 2011;113(5):965–968.
14. Ramsay JG, Rappaport BA. SmartTots: a multidisciplinary effort to determine anesthetic safety in young children. *Anesth Analg*. 2011;113(5):963–964.
15. Ikonomidou C, Bosch F, Miksa M, et al.. Blockade of NMDA receptors and apoptotic neurodegeneration in the developing brain. *Science*. 1999;283:70–74.
16. Ikonomidou C, Bittigau P, Ishimaru MJ, et al.. Ethanol-induced apoptotic neurodegeneration and fetal alcohol syndrome. *Science*. 2000;287:1056–1060.

17. Jevtovic-Todorovic V, Hartman RE, Izumi Y, et al. Early exposure to common anesthetic agents causes widespread neurodegeneration in the developing rat brain and persistent learning deficits. *J Neurosci.* 2003;23:876–824.

18. Fredriksson A, Archer T, Alm H, Gordh T, Eriksson P. Neurofunctional deficits and potentiated apoptosis by neonatal NMDA antagonist administration. *Behav Brain Res.* 2004;153:367–376.

19. Young C, Jevtovic-Todorovic V, Qin YQ, et al. Potential of ketamine and midazolam, individually or in combination, to induce apoptotic neurodegeneration in the infant mouse brain. *Br J Pharmacol.* 2005;146:189–197.

20. Fredriksson A, Ponten E, Gordh T, Eriksson P. Neonatal exposure to a combination of N-methyl-d-aspartate and γ-aminobutyric acid type A receptor anesthetic agents potentiates apoptotic neurodegeneration and persistent behavioral deficits. *Anesthesiology.* 2007;107:427–436.

21. Nikizad H, Yon JH, Carter LB, Jevtovic-Todorovic V. Early exposure to general anesthesia causes significant neuronal deletion in the developing rat brain. *Ann N Y Acad Sci.* 2007;1122:69–82.

22. Johnson SA, Young C, Olney JW. Isoflurane-induced neuroapoptosis in the developing brain of non-hypoglycemic mice. *J Neurosurg Anesth.* 2008;20:21–28.

23. Cattano D, Young C, Olney JW. Sub-anesthetic doses of propofol induce neuroapoptosis in the infant mouse brain. *Anesth Analg.* 2008;106:1712–1714.

24. Zhang X, Xue Z, Sun A. Subclinical concentration of sevoflurane potentiates neuronal apoptosis in the developing C57BL/6 mouse brain. *Neurosci Lett.* 2008;447:109–114.

25. Satomoto M, Satoh Y, Terui K, et al. Neonatal exposure to sevoflurane induces abnormal social behaviors and deficits in fear conditioning in mice. *Anesthesiology.* 2009;110:628–637.

26. Liang G, Ward C, Peng J, Zhao Y, Huang B, Wei H. Isoflurane causes greater neurodegeneration than an equivalent exposure of sevoflurane in the developing brain of neonatal mice. *Anesthesiology.* 2010;112:1325–1334.

27. Istaphanous GK, Howard J, Nan X, et al. Comparison of the neuroapoptotic properties of equipotent anesthetic concentrations of desflurane, isoflurane, or sevoflurane in neonatal mice. *Anesthesiology.* 2011;114:578–587.

28. Rizzi S, Carter LB, Ori C, Jevtovic-Todorovic V. Clinical anesthesia causes permanent damage to the fetal guinea pig brain. *Brain Pathol.* 2008;18:198–210.

29. Slikker W Jr, Zou X, Hotchkiss CE, et al. Ketamine-induced neuronal cell death in the perinatal rhesus monkey. *Toxicol Sci.* 2007;98:145–158.

30. Zou X, Patterson TA, Divine RL, et al. Prolonged exposure to ketamine increases neurodegeneration in the developing monkey brain. *Int J Dev Neurosci.* 2009;27:727–731.

31. Brambrink AM, Evers AS, Avidan MS, et al. Isoflurane-induced neuroapoptosis in the neonatal rhesus macaque brain. *Anesthesiology.* 2010;112:834–841.

32. Brambrink AM, Back SA, Avidan MS, Creeley CE, Olney JW. Ketamine and isoflurane anesthesia triggers neuronal and glial apoptosis in the neonatal macaque. Abstract presented at: American Society of Anesthesiologists Annual Meeting, San Diego, CA, October 16-20, 2010.

33. Zou X, Liu F, Zhang X, et al. Inhalation anesthetic-induced neuronal damage in the developing rhesus monkey. *Neurotoxicol Teratol.* 2011;33:592–597.

34. Paule MG, Li M, Zou X, et al. Ketamine anesthesia during the first week of life can cause long-lasting cognitive deficits in rhesus monkeys. *Neurotoxicol Teratol.* 2011;33:220–230.

35. Brambrink AM, Evers AS, Avidan MS, et al. Ketamine-induced neuroapoptosis in the fetal and neonatal rhesus macaque brain. *Anesthesiology.* 2012;116:372–384.

36. Brambrink AM, Back SA, Riddle A, et al. Isoflurane-induced apoptosis of oligodendrocytes in the neonatal primate brain. *Ann Neurol.* 2012;72:525–535.

37. Anand KJS, Soriano SG. Anesthetic agents and the immature brain: are these toxic or therapeutic? *Anesthesiology.* 2004;101:527–530.

38. Soriano SG, Loepke AW. Let's not throw the baby out with the bath water: potential neurotoxicity of anesthetic drugs in infants and children. *J Neurosurg Anesthesiol.* 2005;17:207–209.

39. Anand KJ. Anesthetic neurotoxicity in newborns. Should we change clinical practice? *Anesthesiology.* 2007;107:2–4.

40. DiMaggio CJ, Sun L, Kakavouli A, Byrne MW, Li G. A retrospective cohort study of the association of anesthesia and hermia repair surgery with behavioral and developmental disorders in young children. *J Neurosurg Anesthesiol.* 2009;21:286–291.

41. DiMaggio CJ, Sun LS, Li G. Early childhood exposure to anesthesia and risk of developmental and behavioral disorders in a sibling birth cohort. *Anesth Analg.* 2011;113:1143–1151.

42. Wilder RT, Flick RP, Sprung J, et al. Early exposure to anesthesia and learning disabilities in a population-based birth cohort. *Anesthesiology.* 2009;110:796–804.

43. Flick RP, Katusic SK, Colligan RC, et al. Cognitive and behavioral outcomes after early exposure to anesthesia and surgery. *Pediatrics.* 2011;128(5):e1053–e1061..

44. Sprung J, Flick RP, Katusic SK, et al. Attention-deficit/hyperactivity disorder after early exposure to procedures requiring general anesthesia. *Mayo Clin Proc.* 2012;87(2):120–129.

45. Thomas JJ, Choi JY, Bayman EO, Kimble KK, Todd MM, Block RI. Does anesthesia exposure in infancy affect academic performance in childhood? Poster presented at: IARS and SAFEKIDS International Science Symposium "Anesthetic-Induced Neonatal Neuronal Injury," International Anesthesia Research Society Annual Meeting; March 20, 2010; Hawaii; poster session abstract ISS-A4. Available at www.IARS.org.

46. Kalkman CJ, Peelen LM, deJong TP, Sinnema G, Moons KG. Behavior and development in children and age at time of first anesthetic exposure: *Anesthesiology.* 2009;110:805–812.

47. Hansen TG, Pedersen JK, Henneberg SW, et al. Academic performance in adolescence after inguinal hernia repair in infancy: a nationwide cohort study. *Anesthesiology.* 2011;114(5):1076–1085.

48. Bartels M, Althoff RR, Boomsma DI. Anesthesia and cognitive performance in children: no evidence for a causal relationship. *Twin Res Hum Genet.* 2009;12(3):246–253.

49. Davidson AJ, McCann ME, Morton NS, Myles PS. Anesthesia and outcome after neonatal surgery: the role for randomized trials. *Anesthesiology.* 2008;109(6):941–944.

50. Sun LS, Li G, Dimaggio C, et al.; Coinvestigators of the Pediatric Anesthesia Neurodevelopment Assessment (PANDA) Research Network. Anesthesia and neurodevelopment in children: time for an answer? *Anesthesiology.* 2008;109(5):757–761.

51. McCann M, Davidson A, Morton N, Frawley G, Hunt R, et al. An update on progress of the multi-site RCT comparing regional and general anesthesia for effects on neurodevelopmental outcome and apnea in infants—the GAS Study. Poster presented at: IARS and SAFEKIDS International Science Symposium "Anesthetic-Induced Neonatal Neuronal Injury," International Anesthesia Research Society Annual Meeting; March 20, 2010; Hawaii; Poster Session Abstract ISS-A14. Available at www.IARS.org.

52. Sun LS, Byrne M, Forde A, Li G, DiMaggio C, Rauh V, Kakavouli A; co-investigators of the PANDA Research Network. PANDA Study: status update. Poster presented at: IARS and SAFEKIDS International Science Symposium "Anesthetic-Induced Neonatal Neuronal Injury," International Anesthesia Research Society Annual Meeting; March 20, 2010; Hawaii; Poster Session Abstract ISS-A15. Available at www.IARS.org.

53. Kodama M, Satoh Y, Otsubo Y, et al. Neonatal desflurane exposure induces more robust neuroapoptosis than do isoflurane and sevoflurane and impairs working memory. *Anesthesiology.* 2011;115(5):979–991.

54. Cattano D, Straiko MMW, Olney JW. Chloral hydrate induces and lithium prevents neuroapoptosis in the infant mouse brain. Paper

presented at: American Society of Anesthesiologists Annual Meeting; Oralndo, October 2008. Abstract #A315. Avaliable at www.asaabstracts.com.

55. Bittigau P, Sifringer M, Genz K, et al. Antiepileptic drugs and apoptotic neurodegeneration in the developing brain. *Proc Nat Acad Sci.* 2002;99:15089–15094.

56. Creeley CE, Yuede CM, Olney JW. Caffeine potentiates neuroapoptosis induced in the infant mouse brain by alcohol. Society for Neuroscience, 2010; abstr. no. 842.24. Available at www.SFN.com.

57. Olney JW, Creeley CE, Yuede CM. Caffeine augments neuroapoptosis induced in the infant mouse brain by isoflurane. Paper presented at: IARS and SAFEKIDS International Science Symposium "Anesthetic-Induced Neonatal Neuronal Injury," International Anesthesiology Research Society Annual Meeting; March 20, 2010. Available at www.IARS.org.

58. Olney JW, Creeley CE, Yuede CM. Caffeine potentiates neuroapoptosis induced in the infant mouse brain by isoflurane. Paper presented at: American Society of Anesthesiologists Annual Meeting; San Diego, CA, October 2010. Available at www.asaabstracts.com.

59. Olney JW, Creeley CE, Yuede CM. Caffeine potentiates diazepam-induced neuroapoptosis in the developing mouse brain. Society for Neuroscience; San Diego, CA, November 2010; abstr. no. 842.17. Available at www.SFN.com.

60. Natarajan G, Botica M-L, Thomas R, Aranda JV. Therapeutic drug monitoring for caffeine in preterm neonates: an unnecessary exercise? *Pediatrics.* 2007;119:936–940.

61. Charles BG, Townsend SR, Steer PA, Flenady VJ, Gray PH, Shearman A. Caffeine citrate treatment for extremely premature infants with apnea: population pharmacokinetics, absolute bioavailability, and implications for therapeutic drug monitoring. *Ther Drug Monit.* 2008;30:709–716.

62. Dobbing J, Sands J. The brain growth spurt in various mammalian species. *Early Hum Dev.* 1979;3:79–84.

63. Rice D, Barone S Jr. Critical periods of vulnerability for the developing nervous system: evidence from human and animal models. *Environ Health Perspect.* 2000;108(S3):511–533.

64. Farber NB, Creeley CE, Olney JW. Alcohol-induced neuroapoptosis in the fetal macaque brain. *Neurobiol Dis.* 2010;40(1):200–206.

65. Wozniak DF, Hartman RE, Boyle MP, et al. Apoptotic neurodegeneration induced by ethanol in neonatal mice is associated with profound learning/memory deficits in juveniles followed by progressive functional recovery in adults. *Neurobiol Dis.* 2004;17:403–414.

66. Zhu C, Gao J, Karlsson N, et al. Isoflurane anesthesia induced persistent, progressive memory impairment, caused a loss of neural stem cells, and reduced neurogenesis in young, but not adult, rodents. *J Cereb Blood Flow Metab.* 2010;30(5):1017–1030.

67. Shih J, May LD, Gonzalez HE, et al. Delayed environmental enrichment reverses sevoflurane-induced memory impairment in rats. *Anesthesiology.* 2012;116(3):586–602.

68. Rizzi S, Ori C, Jevtovic-Todorovic V. Timing versus duration: determinants of anesthesia-induced developmental apoptosis in the young mammalian brain. *Ann N Y Acad Sci.* 2010;1199:43–51.

69. Mattson SN, Riley EP, Sowell ER, Jernigan TL, Sobel DF, Jones KL. A decrease in the size of the basal ganglia in children with fetal alcohol syndrome. *Alcohol Clin Exp Res.* 1996;20:1088–1093.

70. Riley EP, McGee CL. Fetal alcohol spectrum disorders: an overview with emphasis on changes in brain and behavior. *Exp Biol Med.* 2005;230:357–365.

71. Ikonomidou C, Scheer I, Wilhelm T, et al. Brain morphology alterations in the basal ganglia and the hypothalamus following prenatal exposure to antiepileptic drugs. *Eur J Paediatr Neurol.* 2007;11:297–301.

72. Zhou ZW, Shu Y, Li M, Guo X, Pac-Soo C, Maze M, Ma D. The glutaminergic, GABAergic, dopaminergic but not cholinergic neurons are susceptible to anaesthesia-induced cell death in the rat developing brain. *Neuroscience.* 2011;174:64–70.

73. Olney JW, Young C, Qin Y-Q, Dikranian K, Farber NB. Ethanol-induced developmental glioapoptosis in mice and monkeys. Presented at the Society for Neuroscience Annual Meeting; Washington, DC, November 2005; abstr. #916.7. Available at www.SFN.com.

74. Head BP, Patel HH, Niesman IR, Drummond JC, Roth DM, Patel PM. Inhibition of p75 neurotrophin receptor attenuates isoflurane-mediated neuronal apoptosis in the neonatal central nervous system. *Anesthesiology.* 2009;110(4):813–825.

75. Lemkuil BP, Head BP, Pearn ML, Patel HH, Drummond JC, Patel PM. Isoflurane neurotoxicity is mediated by p75NTR-RhoA activation and actin depolymerization. *Anesthesiology.* 2011;114(1):49–57.

76. De Roo M, Klauser P, Briner A, et al. Anesthetics rapidly promote synaptogenesis during a critical period of brain development. *PLoS One.* 2009;4(9):e7043.

77. Briner A, De Roo M, Dayer A, Muller D, Habre W, Vutskits L. Volatile anesthetics rapidly increase dendritic spine density in the rat medial prefrontal cortex during synaptogenesis. *Anesthesiology.* 2010;112(3):546–556.

78. Briner A, Nikonenko I, De Roo M, Dayer A, Muller D, Vutskits L. Developmental Stage-dependent persistent impact of propofol anesthesia on dendritic spines in the rat medial prefrontal cortex. *Anesthesiology.* 2011;115(2):282–293.

79. Stratmann G, Sall JW, May LD, et al. Isoflurane differentially affects neurogenesis and long-term neurocognitive function in 60-day-old and 7-day-old rats. *Anesthesiology.* 2009;110(4):834–848.

80. Zhu C, Gao J, Karlsson N, et al. Isoflurane anesthesia induced persistent, progressive memory impairment, caused a loss of neural stem cells, and reduced neurogenesis in young, but not adult, rodents. *J Cereb Blood Flow Metab.* 2010;30:1017–1030.

81. Klintsova AY, Helfer JL, Calizo LH, Dong WK, Goodlett CR, Greenough WT. Persistent impairment of hippocampal neurogenesis in young adult rats following early postnatal alcohol exposure. *Alcohol Clin Exp Res.* 2007;31:2073–2082.

82. Stefovska VG, Uckermann O, Czuczwar M, et al. Sedative and anticonvulsant drugs suppress postnatal neurogenesis. *Ann Neurol.* 2008;64:434–445.

83. Dikranian K, Ishimaru MJ, Tenkova T, et al. Apoptosis in the in vivo mammalian forebrain. *Neurobiol Dis.* 2001;8:359–379.

84. Dikranian K, Qin YQ, Labruyere J, Nemmers B, Olney JW. Ethanol-induced neuroapoptosis in the developing rodent cerebellum and related brain stem structures. *Dev Brain Res.* 2005;155:1–13.

85. Tenkova T, Young C, Dikranian K, Olney JW. Ethanol-induced apoptosis in the visual system during synaptogenesis. *Invest Ophthalmol Vis Sci.* 2003;44:2809–2817.

86. Young C, Straiko MM, Johnson SA, Creeley C, Olney JW. Ethanol causes and lithium prevents neuroapoptosis and suppression of pERK in the infant mouse brain. *Neurobiol Dis.* 2008;31:355–360.

87. Straiko MMW, Young C, Cattano D, et al. Lithium protects against anesthesia-induced developmental neuroapoptosis. *Anesthesiology.* 2009;110:662–668.

88. Sanders RD, Sun P, Patel S, Li M, Maze M, Ma D. Dexmedetomidine provides cortical neuroprotection: impact on anaesthetic-induced neuroapoptosis in the rat developing brain. *Acta Anaesthesiol Scand.* 2010;54:710–716.

89. Yon JH, Carter LB, Jevtovic-Todorovic V. Melatonin reduces the severity of anesthesia-induced apoptotic neurodegeneration in the developing rat brain. *Neurobiol Dis.* 2006;21:522–530.

90. Ma D, Williamson P, Januszewski A, et al. Xenon mitigates isoflurane-induced neuronal apoptosis in the developing rodent brain. *Anesthesiology.* 2007;106(4):746–753.

91. Sanders RD, Xu J, Shu Y, et al. Dexmedetomidine attenuates isoflurane-induced neurocognitive impairment in neonatal rats. *Anesthesiology.* 2009;110(5):1077–1085.

92. Sanders RD, Sun P, Patel S, Li M, Maze M, Ma D. Dexmedetomidine provides cortical neuroprotection: impact on anaesthetic-induced neuroapoptosis in the rat developing brain. *Acta Anaesthesiol Scand.* 2010;54(6):710–716.

93. Shu Y, Patel SM, Pac-Soo C, et al. Xenon pretreatment attenuates anesthetic-induced apoptosis in the developing brain in comparison with nitrous oxide and hypoxia. *Anesthesiology.* 2010;113(2):360–368.

94. Young C, Klocke J, Tenkova T, et al. Ethanol-induced neuronal apoptosis in the in vivo developing mouse brain is BAX dependent. *Cell Death Differ.* 2003;10:1148–1155.

95. Jiang H, Huang Y, Xu H, Sun Y, Han N, Li QF. Hypoxia inducible factor-1α is involved in the neurodegeneration induced by isoflurane in the brain of neonatal rats. *J Neurochem.* 2012;120(3):453–460.

96. Olney JW, Tenkova T, Dikranian K, et al. Ethanol-induced caspase-3 activation in the in vivo developing mouse brain. *Neurobiol Dis.* 2002;9:205–219.

97. Young C, Roth KA, Klocke BJ, et al. Role of caspase-3 in ethanol-induced developmental neurodegeneration. *Neurobiol Dis.* 2005;20:608–614.

98. Pearn ML, Hu Y, Niesman IR, et al. Propofol neurotoxicity is mediated by p75 neurotrophin receptor activation. *Anesthesiology.* 2012;116(2):352–361.

99. Yon JH, Daniel-Johnson J, Carter LB, Jevtovic-Todorovic V. Anesthesia induces suicide in the developing rat brain via the intrinsic and extrinsic apoptotic pathways. *Neuroscience.* 2005;135:815–827.

100. Lu LX, Yon JH, Carter LB, Jevtovic-Todorovic V. General anesthesia activates BDNF-dependent neuroapoptosis in the developing rat brain. *Apoptosis.* 2006;11:1603–1615.

101. Zhao YL, Xiang Q, Shi QY, et al. GABAergic excitotoxicity injury of the immature hippocampal pyramidal neurons' exposure to isoflurane. *Anesth Analg.* 2011;113(5):1152–1160.

102. Ben-Ari Y, Gaiarsa JL, Tyzio R, Khazipov R. GABA: a pioneer transmitter that excites immature neurons and generates primitive oscillations. *Physiol Rev.* 2007;87(4):1215–1284.

103. Yamada J, Okabe A, Toyoda H, Kilb W, Luhmann HJ, Fukuda A. Cl- uptake promoting depolarizing GABA actions in immature rat neocortical neurones is mediated by NKCC1. *J Physiol.* 2004;557(Pt 3):829–841.

104. Rivera C, Voipio J, Payne JA, et al. The K+/Cl- co-transporter KCC2 renders GABA hyperpolarizing during neuronal maturation. *Nature.* 1999;397(6716):251–255.

105. Zou X, Sadovova N, Patterson TA, et al. The effects of L-carnitine on the combination of, inhalation anesthetic-induced developmental, neuronal apoptosis in the rat frontal cortex. *Neuroscience.* 2008;151(4):1053–1065.

106. Edwards DA, Shah HP, Cao W, Gravenstein N, Seubert CN, Martynyuk AE. Bumetanide alleviates epileptogenic and neurotoxic effects of sevoflurane in neonatal rat brain. *Anesthesiology.* 2010;112(3):567–575.

107. Tsuchimoto T, Ueki M, Miki T, Morishita J, Maekawa N. Erythropoietin attenuates isoflurane-induced neurodegeneration and learning deficits in the developing mouse brain. *Paediatr Anaesth.* 2011;21(12):1209–1213.

108. Creeley CE, Olney JW. The young: neuroapoptosis induced by anesthetics and what to do about it. *Anesth Analg.* 2010;110(2):442–448.

109. Makaryus R, Lee H, Yu M, et al. The metabolomic profile during isoflurane anesthesia differs from propofol anesthesia in the live rodent brain. *J Cereb Blood Flow Metab.* 2011;31(6):1432–1442.

110. DiMaggio C, Sun LS, Ing C, Li G. Pediatric anesthesia and neurodevelopmental impairments: a Bayesian meta-analysis. *J Neurosurg Anesthesiol.* 2012: 24(4):376–81.

111. Wang C. Advanced pre-clinical research approaches and models to studying pediatric anesthetic neurotoxicity. *Front Neurol* 2012;3:142.

112. Jevtovic-Todorovic V, Boscolo A, Sanchez V, Lunardi N. Anesthesia-induced developmental neurodegeneration: the role of neuronal organelles. *Front Neurol* 2012;3:141.

2.

DELIRIUM

Elizabeth L. Whitlock, Michael S. Avidan, and Sharon K. Inouye

INTRODUCTION TO THE CLINICAL PROBLEM

The word *delirium* derives from the Latin *deliriare*, which may be translated as "to go off the furrow" or ploughed track in a field. Delirium has long been recognized as a complication of surgical or medical illness; however, until the last few decades, it received little attention in the medical literature. Delirium is defined in the *Diagnostic and Statistical Manual of Mental Disorders*, 4th edition (DSM-IV), as an acute, fluctuating disturbance of consciousness with impairment of attention and cognition that results from a medical condition. The biochemical pathophysiology of delirium has been recently reviewed[1]; it has been hypothesized to be a manifestation of abnormalities in virtually every neurotransmitter system, though cholinergic transmission is particularly implicated. Delirium may complicate the postoperative course both early, as anesthetic and supportive medications are metabolized, and late, on the hospital ward or intensive care unit (ICU). Within the last two decades, the remarkably high prevalence of delirium in critical care and geriatric care settings has been established, and the prevention, treatment, use as a prognostic tool, and potential sequelae of this complication are all being actively investigated. It has long been appreciated that acute organ dysfunction, such as renal impairment or respiratory insufficiency, can occur postoperatively or as a component of critical illness. Delirium might be a manifestation of acute brain dysfunction.

INCIDENCE, PREVALENCE, AND OUTCOMES

Incidence rates of postoperative delirium range widely depending on the type and invasiveness of surgery and the patient population on whom the surgeries are performed (Table 2.1). Studies of unselected adult patients in the postoperative recovery area have found incidence rates of approximately 10%.[2] In contrast, for those in whom surgery is complicated by critical illness, delirium prevalence in the surgical ICU approaches 75%.[3] Following cardiac surgery, postoperative (typically ICU) delirium rates may be as low as 16% in younger patients undergoing elective surgery.[4] Not surprisingly, however, studies including or focusing on the elderly and nonelective (emergent) cases have typically found higher rates of approximately 40–50%.[5,6] Another well-studied population is that of elderly patients undergoing elective or urgent orthopedic surgery; rates range from under 20% after elective surgery[7] to 30–40% following urgent surgery to repair a hip fracture.[8,9] Rates of postoperative delirium following specific surgical procedures were recently reviewed by Rudolph and Marcantonio.[10]

Many observational studies have clearly shown an association between postoperative delirium and subsequent cognitive and functional morbidity and in-hospital and out-of-hospital mortality. A very large study of patients undergoing coronary artery bypass grafting demonstrated a hazard ratio for death, adjusted for perioperative and vascular risk factors, in patients suffering postoperative delirium

Table 2.1 OVERVIEW OF DELIRIUM RATES IN DIFFERENT CLINICAL CONTEXTS

TYPE	STUDY (YEAR)	POPULATION	RATE	DETECTION METHOD
All patients	Radtke (2010)[2]	Recovery room after elective general anesthesia	9.9%	Nu-DESC
Surgical ICU	Pandharipande (2008)[3]	Surgical ICU	73%	CAM-ICU
		Trauma ICU	67%	
Ocular	Milstein (2002) in Rudolph (2011)[10]	Cataract	4.4%	CRS
Head and neck	Weed (1995) in Rudolph (2011)[10]	Major head and neck	17%	Not stated
Cardiac	Kazmierski (2010)[4]	Cardiac surgery with CPB	Age <60: 16.3% Age ≥60: 24.7%	DSM-IV
	Rudolph (2010)[5]	Patients >60 undergoing elective or urgent cardiac surgery	43%	CAM
Abdominal	Marcantonio (1994) and Olin (2005) in Rudolph (2011)[10]	Abdominal surgery	5–51%	CAM
	Kaneko (1997) and Mann (2000) in Rudolph (2011)[10]	Patients >70 undergoing abdominal surgery	17–25%	DSM-III
Vascular	Marcantonio (1994), Schneider (2002), Bohner (2003), and Benoit (2005) in Rudolph (2011)[10]	Abdominal aortic aneurysm repair	33–54%	CAM or DSM-IV
	Schneider (2002) and Bohner (2003) in Rudolph (2011)[10]	Peripheral vascular	30–48%	DSM-IV
Orthopedic	Fisher (1995)[7]	Patients >60 undergoing elective orthopedic procedures	17.5%	CAM
	Marcantonio (2000)[8] and Lee (2011)[9]	Patients >65 undergoing emergent hip fracture repair	30.2–41%	CAM

ABBREVIATIONS: CAM: Confusion Assessment Method; CPB: cardiopulmonary bypass; CRS: Confusion Rating Scale; DSM-IV: *Diagnostic and Statistical Manual of Mental Disorders*, 4th ed.; Nu-DESC: Nursing Delirium Screening Scale.

of 1.65 (95% confidence interval 1.38–1.97), which persisted up to 10 years following surgery.[11] Not limited to cardiac surgical patients,[12] increased risk of death following postoperative delirium has also been demonstrated in elderly patients following orthopedic[8,13] and abdominal[14] surgery. ICU and/or hospital length of stay are also significantly longer for patients with postoperative delirium.[14,15]

Postoperative delirium is also associated with increased rates of subsequent functional decline in the elderly. Patients with postoperative delirium are twice as likely to suffer declines in ability to complete basic and/or instrumental activities of daily living,[5,8,12] are two to three times as likely to be discharged to a setting other than home (e.g., nursing home),[8,14] and are at least twice as likely to need long-term care.[13,16] Cognitive outcomes are also worse in patients with postoperative delirium, which is independently associated with increased rates of subjective memory decline,[12,16] cognitive impairment, and/or dementia.[13,16]

These many important relationships have led to estimates of the increased health care costs associated with a diagnosis of delirium. A small study published in 2001 found that hospital direct and indirect costs, as well as ward nursing costs,

increased by 20–25% for patients with delirium after elective noncardiac surgery.[15] A broader look at increased costs has only been published for nonsurgical patients. One study of elderly patients (aged greater than 70 years) showed that for the first year following a diagnosis of incident delirium associated with a medical—not surgical—illness, adjusted average costs for patients with delirium were 2 to 2.5 times the cost for those who were nondelirious. This resulted in an additional $16,000 to $64,000 in costs per person per year, which, if extended across the estimated rate of delirium across the U.S. health care system, implies costs of $38 to $152 billion (2005 U.S. dollars) per year.[17] The study, which excluded patients with delirium or known dementia at baseline, offers the best current estimate of the potential costs associated with delirium—an entity that was thought for many centuries to be of little clinical significance.

RISK FACTORS

Risk factors for postoperative delirium reflect a complex interplay between patient, pre- and intraoperative care, and postoperative factors. This framework proves useful when predicting which patients are at highest risk for delirium—thus allowing targeted delivery of interventions—and predicting which interventions might prove useful in vulnerable patients.

Knowledge of nonmodifiable patient-related factors allows targeted screening and preventative interventions in those most vulnerable to postoperative delirium. Many patient factors—including advanced age,[2,4,5,8,18] preoperative cognitive impairment or dementia,[2,4–6,8,18] baseline functional impairment,[5,8,14] and pre-existing comorbid medical illness[5,8,14]—are common to virtually all studies of delirium risk factors in both the surgical and medical literature. Certain risk factors, including dementia or cognitive impairment, advanced age, low educational attainment, alcohol abuse, prior stroke or transient ischemic attack,[6,18] and pre-existing depression,[2,4,6,18] have informed a theory that delirium risk is in part predicated on a patient's "cognitive reserve," summarized in a review by Jones and colleagues.[19]

Another useful indicator of postoperative delirium risk is low serum albumin concentration.[6,18,20] Albumin provides a surrogate for nutritional status, which may in turn be related to functional status and cognitive reserve. It also plays an essential role in drug distribution; with reduced albumin, the free fraction of a protein-binding drug may be elevated (leading to increased drug effect) early after its administration. There may be a relationship between the duration of fluid restriction preoperatively and postoperative delirium[21]; albumin also plays an important role in the maintenance of intravascular fluid homeostasis. Furthermore, with its role as a negative acute-phase reactant, low albumin may reflect systemic inflammation, another hypothesized contributor to delirium risk.

While nonmodifiable patient factors are useful for baseline risk-stratification, modifiable aspects of perioperative care suggest potential avenues for reducing delirium incidence. Postoperative delirium has been associated with the use of anticholinergics (which may include muscle relaxants and gastrointestinal antispasmodics) and psychotropic medications, particularly benzodiazepines but also antiepileptics and antidepressants. Meperidine has been associated with postoperative delirium, and fentanyl[2,3] and tramadol[14] less strongly so; however, undertreated postoperative pain also increases delirium risk. Many studies have shown an association between intraoperative red blood cell transfusions[18] or surrogates of transfusion (e.g., preoperative anemia[2] or greater intraoperative blood loss[20]) and the development of postoperative delirium; this may reflect operative invasiveness and/or the effect of inflammatory mediators.

Another interesting avenue of recent research is the relationship between intraoperative hemodynamic variables and subsequent delirium. Observational studies have shown increased risk of delirium with low regional pre-[22,23] and intraoperative[23] regional cerebral oxygen saturation and postoperative hypoxemia.[4] Intraoperative hypotension is also associated with increased risk.[20] While a randomized trial of intraoperative hypoxemia would likely prove ethically infeasible, a small randomized trial of increased perfusion pressure during cardiopulmonary bypass found a lower rate of delirium when mean perfusion pressure was maintained at 80–90 mmHg compared with standard of care (60–70 mmHg).[24] Blood pressure, cerebral perfusion pressure, cerebral oxygenation, and vascular risk factors interact in a complex manner and have often been shown to be associated with postoperative delirium, particularly in cardiac surgical populations.[18] The contribution of potentially modifiable aspects of intraoperative physiology to postoperative delirium deserves further research.

Many environmental factors have been implicated as potentially contributing to delirium risk, although they have not been as vigorously pursued in the surgical literature. These include unfamiliar environments, sensory impairment (i.e., patient's lack of hearing aids or glasses), sleep–wake cycle disturbances commonly resulting from medical procedures or examinations that take place during sleeping hours, disorientation to time from poor access to natural light and/or limited availability of or difficulty reading clocks, use of restraints, and use of a urinary catheter. These risk factors represent important areas targeted in the multicomponent delirium prevention strategies, described further below.

PREVENTION AND TREATMENT

Strategies for prevention and treatment of adult delirium are presented below, stratified by pharmacologic and non-pharmacologic approaches.

NONPHARMACOLOGIC

For perhaps a decade, the only known effective preventative strategy was the Hospital Elder Life Program (HELP) multicomponent intervention demonstrated by Inouye and colleagues in 1999 in a population of 852 medical inpatients. The intervention, which targeted patients at least 70 years old who were free of delirium and dementia at baseline but judged to be at moderate or high risk for delirium, reduced ward delirium rates from 15% in the usual-care group to 9.9% and significantly reduced total number of delirium episodes and delirium days.[25] The HELP model is implemented by an interdisciplinary team that conducts interventions in the domains of cognition, sleep, mobility, vision and hearing adaptations, and maintenance of nutrition and hydration.

Subsequent studies have demonstrated the benefits of HELP for greater reductions of delirium,[26,27] reduction of cognitive and functional decline,[28] length of hospital stay,[26,27,29] hospital falls,[29] sitter use,[29] and institutionalization.[29,30] Hospital cost savings of $1000 per patient have been demonstrated[26,31] as well as savings of $10,000 per patient for long-term nursing home costs.[30] Caplan et al. demonstrated savings of $121,425 per year in sitter costs with a HELP model in Australia.[29] The HELP model is now implemented in hundreds of hospitals around the world (more information is available at www.hospitalelderlifeprogram.org).

An adapted version of HELP, which focused on three protocols (early mobilization, nutrition, and reorientation/therapeutic activities) was assessed in elderly patients following elective abdominal surgery. In this small before-after study of 179 surgical patients, the modified HELP program reduced delirium rates (from 17% to 0%) and slowed decline in functional and nutritional status in these elderly patients. The simplicity of this version will enhance the feasibility of implementation; however, further evaluation with concurrent controls is indicated before widespread adoption.[32] Similarly, involving a geriatrician in the care of elderly patients after hip fracture repair through a proactive geriatric consultation model reduced delirium rates from 50% to 32%.[33] Optimizing the patients' environment, mobility, nutrition, and medication regimen is the most effective method of reducing delirium rates, carries the lowest risk of harm, and should be considered for every geriatric patient (if not every unselected patient) in the perioperative setting.

Approaches to minimize sedation or anesthesia are increasingly recognized as important to decreasing the incidence and duration of delirium. Interesting hypotheses have been advanced that implicate cerebral connectivity and inhibitory tone in the development of delirium.[34] These hypotheses are particularly important to anesthesiologists, as anesthetic drugs fundamentally alter connectivity and inhibitory tone, ostensibly producing a temporary effect that allows for their return to normal after the conclusion of anesthesia. A handful of studies have been designed to look at the effect of regional anesthesia (RA) with sedation compared with general anesthesia (GA). A meta-analysis of fairly heterogeneous randomized controlled trials of GA versus other anesthetic methods for a variety of operations found no significantly increased rate of postoperative delirium with GA.[35] Subsequently, a trial was conducted in which participants undergoing hip fracture surgery were randomized to either light sedation (bispectral index [BIS] > 80) or deep sedation (BIS target = 50) with propofol. All procedures were performed with spinal anesthesia. The authors demonstrated a significantly increased rate of delirium with GA-like level of sedation: 40% of the patients receiving deep sedation had an episode of delirium, compared with only 19% of those receiving light sedation.[36] Theoretically, deep anesthesia resulting in burst suppression or persistent suppression might render the brain even more susceptible to postoperative delirium. Unlike other electroencephalographic patterns during GA, burst suppression and persistent suppression do not occur during physiological sleep. Burst suppression has been shown to occur more frequently in patients with comorbidities, such as cardiac disease, and has been associated with increased 6-month mortality when it has been observed in critically ill patients. Further well-designed trials in this area will be essential to resolve the existing debate; certainly there is excellent theoretical justification for minimizing the administration of drugs known to affect cerebral connectivity and inhibitory tone in patients who have a high vulnerability to delirium.

PHARMACOLOGIC

Trials investigating pharmacologic prevention and treatment of delirium have been hampered by small sample sizes, heterogeneous patient populations, and variability in screening methods.

Cholinesterase inhibitors, despite their promise given that relative acetylcholine deficiency seems to be implicated in the pathogenesis of delirium, have been disappointing. Three small trials of donepezil for delirium prevention have shown no difference versus placebo after elective hip replacement or hip fracture surgery. A small cardiac surgical study showed no difference in delirium when prophylactic rivastigmine was given; subsequently, a trial of rivastigmine in the treatment of ICU delirium was halted early because of higher mortality in the rivastigmine group than in the placebo group.

More promising are the typical and atypical antipsychotics, which are the mainstay of pharmacologic delirium treatment in most clinical situations. Two studies have evaluated the use of prophylactic haloperidol. One evaluated 1.5 mg haloperidol versus placebo per day in 430 elderly patients undergoing hip replacement and demonstrated no significant difference in delirium incidence but significantly shorter duration of delirium and hospital length of stay in the haloperidol group compared with the placebo group.[37] These results must be interpreted with caution, since the Delirium Rating Scale used for assessment of severity and duration tends to be overly dependent on hyperactive delirium symptoms, which would tend to be suppressed by haloperidol (with potential conversion to an unrecognized hypoactive delirium). In a more recent study, elderly patients admitted to the ICU after noncardiac surgery were randomized to receive intravenous haloperidol 0.5 mg bolus followed by 0.1 mg/h infusion for 12 hours. The haloperidol group experienced a significant reduction in delirium incidence (15.3% versus 23.2%), longer time to onset of delirium and more delirium-free days, and shorter median ICU stay with no major adverse events.[38] These findings represent the most successful pharmacologic prevention strategies to date. Importantly, no study of surgical patients has both successfully prevented the development of delirium and demonstrated a decrease in the morbidity (e.g., decline in functional or cognitive status) with which it is associated. Future pharmacologic prevention studies should focus on these more clinically relevant outcomes.

GUIDELINES AND RECOMMENDATIONS

There are no guidelines on the prevention or management of postoperative delirium specifically. However, many patient-centric risk factors for postoperative and medical delirium overlap significantly, and many interventions shown to be effective in medical delirium are similarly effective in postoperative delirium. Thus, the best guidance comes from national publications that treat delirium—regardless of its medical or surgical antecedents—as a multifactorial disease best addressed by a common pathway of preventative and therapeutic maneuvers.

Varying guidelines have been published by public and private health care organizations since the late 1990s. Most recently, guidelines for the prevention, diagnosis, and management of delirium—of unspecified antecedents—have been published by the United Kingdom's National Institute for Health and Clinical Excellence (NICE) in *DELIRIUM: Diagnosis, Prevention, and Management (Clinical Guideline 103).*[39] This publication is currently the most up-to-date source of evidence-based practice for the prevention and treatment of delirium. An overview of the recommendations is diagrammed in Figure 2.1.

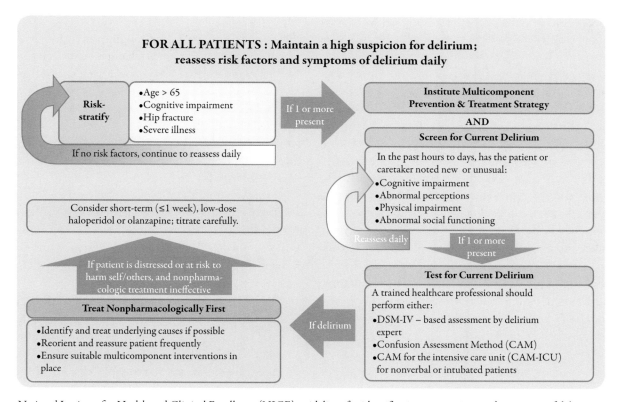

Figure 2.1 National Institute for Health and Clinical Excellence (NICE) guidelines for identification, prevention, and treatment of delirium.

First, NICE recommended maintaining a high suspicion for delirium in any patient who is hospitalized or under long-term care. All patients presenting to a hospital or for long-term care should be assessed for four major risk factors: age greater than 65, pre-existing cognitive impairment, current hip fracture, and severe illness. These risk factors were selected on the basis of a thorough literature review as particularly predictive of increased delirium risk. If any one of these factors is present, the patient is judged to be at risk for delirium and should undergo further assessment. For all patients at risk, a multicomponent intervention package—similar to the Hospital Elder Life Program (HELP)—should be instituted and delivered by an interdisciplinary care team with formal training in prevention of delirium.

The intervention package emphasizes identification and elimination or minimization of factors that can contribute to delirium. To minimize the effects of cognitive impairment and the potential for disorientation, patients should be provided appropriate lighting and time orientation (e.g., a 24-hour clock in critical care settings); frequent reorientation to place, person, and situation; cognitive stimulation; and visits from family and friends, if possible. As dehydration, malnutrition, and constipation can contribute to delirium, appropriate fluid, feeding, and bowel regimens must be used. Expert consultation should be considered in situations where fluid management can be challenging, as in patients with congestive heart failure or renal disease. Patients should be closely monitored for infection, hypoxemia, and pain. As immobility can increase risk, early mobilization after surgery and active range-of-motion exercises should be pursued. Urinary catheters impair mobility, increase infection risk, and have an independent association with delirium; need for urinary catheterization should be reassessed daily. A medication review should be undertaken to minimize medications known to cause delirium in those at risk; in general, the simplest clinically effective regimen should be used, with aggressive refinement of a patient's medication list whenever possible. Reversible sensory impairment—for example, obstruction of the auditory meatus by cerumen—should be addressed; working hearing aids and glasses should be made available to those who need them. Finally, sleep hygiene should be promoted by reducing noise and avoiding medication administration and nursing or medical procedures during sleep hours whenever possible. All of these interventions are part of the HELP model of care.

This multicomponent package should be used for all patients at risk for delirium. Further, those at risk should undergo a second assessment for current symptoms of delirium. Focusing on changes noted in the past few hours or days, patients or caregivers should be asked about new or fluctuating cognitive impairment, abnormal perception (e.g., visual or auditory hallucinations), reduction in physical function, and alteration in social behavior (e.g., unusual social withdrawal, uncooperativeness, changes in mood). If any of those factors are present, further assessment by a reference standard rater (delirium expert) using DSM-IV criteria or the short Confusion Assessment Method (CAM) is recommended. The CAM for the ICU (CAM-ICU) should be reserved for those patients who are nonverbal or intubated in the ICU, since it has been demonstrated to have low sensitivity (<50%) in verbal patients.[40,41] All delirium assessment methods should be carried out by a health care professional trained in these methods. While there are both a long (10-item) and short (4-item) CAM, and both have acceptable sensitivity, the short version has been more widely applied in clinical practice. The short CAM is recommended for routine clinical applications; however, the longer 10-item CAM is preferred where more definitive or research diagnoses for delirium are required. The rationale behind the two-step process recommended by NICE was that a symptoms-based first stage narrows patients to those who may fit within the DSM criteria, while acknowledging that the second-stage diagnostic tests only have low- to moderate-quality evidence available. NICE noted that while these tests in general enjoy high sensitivity, further research should be devoted to development of a highly specific test for delirium.

If delirium is diagnosed, the NICE guidelines emphasize nonpharmacologic treatment (e.g., faithful institution of the multicomponent delirium prevention/treatment model, reorientation strategies, reassurance, and involvement of family and caregivers, if possible). Given the potential for prolonging delirium or adverse effects and the limited evidence to support their use, the NICE guidelines de-emphasize the role of medications in the treatment of delirium. Their use should be limited to patients who are distressed or for those whose delirium poses risk to themselves or others. Short-term (≤1 week), low-dose haloperidol or olanzapine are the two best-supported therapies, although the evidence in surgical patients derives from a single study at high risk of bias; the dose should be carefully titrated to effect. In those with Parkinson's disease or dementia with Lewy bodies, antipsychotics should be used very cautiously, if at all; nonpharmacologic measures are recommended. All studies included in the review for delirium prophylaxis were considered low quality and no pharmacologic prophylaxis could be recommended in any population.

The guidelines also note that, based on review of the evidence and extrapolation to U.K. health care costs, these recommendations are cost-effective. In particular, there is strong evidence that multicomponent interventions are cost-effective in elderly patients undergoing hip fracture repair and for elderly patients at moderate to high risk of delirium admitted to general medical wards. Furthermore, haloperidol and olanzapine are both considered cost-effective treatments; however, the confidence interval around olanzapine is somewhat wider than that for haloperidol.

While the NICE guidelines are the most comprehensive recent review to issue formal recommendations, the Health Services Research and Development Service of the U.S. Department of Veterans Affairs has published a review more recently. In *Delirium: Screening, Prevention, and Diagnosis—A Systematic Review of the Evidence*, no formal recommendations are issued, but avenues for further research are addressed.[42] The authors note the absence of randomized studies demonstrating the effectiveness of screening for delirium in hospitalized patients. A notable weakness of the literature is that there are no data in many populations of patients on the balance of the cost of performing delirium assessments (thus risking misclassification harms) plus the opportunity costs to staff who perform the assessments with the benefits of identifying and treating delirium when it exists. Most studies have been performed in those at elevated risk for delirium and have not been designed to look at harms resulting from misclassification. As reflected in the NICE guidelines, there are no data supporting aggressive delirium screening, prevention, and treatment programs in unselected patients. Furthermore, the multicomponent intervention packages investigated in the literature have not been tested in such a way as to narrow down the contributing effectiveness of individual components; indeed, only small studies have attempted to look at the difference between providing staff education about delirium and usual care alone.

CONCLUSION

Delirium is a relatively common complication of the postoperative course, with rates as low as 10% in unselected populations but approaching 40% in the elderly and 70% in ICU populations. Adult postoperative delirium has been associated repeatedly with morbidity (including subsequent incident dementia, increased hospital length of stay, and subsequent functional decline) and death.

Many risk factors have been identified. Some of the most important ones are those reflecting increased cognitive vulnerability (e.g., advanced age, pre-existing dementia, poor preoperative functional status), a high burden of comorbidities, and low serum albumin. Intraoperative events can also influence delirium risk: several classes of medications, most notably benzodiazepines and anticholinergics, can precipitate delirium, and red blood cell transfusions and markers of abnormal cardiovascular function are also associated with development of postoperative delirium.

The most effective prevention strategies to date have been nonpharmacologic multicomponent interdisciplinary interventions like the Hospital Elder Life Program (HELP), which not only attenuate the functional consequences of postoperative delirium but also reduce in-hospital and out-of-hospital costs. Attempts at pharmacologic prevention have generally been disappointing. Guidelines published by the U.K.'s National Institute for Health and Clinical Excellence (NICE) accordingly emphasize maintaining a high suspicion for delirium, instituting multicomponent prevention strategies for all patients deemed at risk for delirium, and reserving pharmacologic therapy for patients at risk of self-harm.

These recent guidelines and systematic reviews also highlight deficiencies in the literature. Randomized controlled trials of pharmacologic interventions, subcomponents of the successful multicomponent interventions that have been described, and even delirium screening itself in various medical settings will be interesting future directions for the field. Rigorous studies of intraoperative interventions, such as hemodynamic targets, anesthetic techniques, and brain monitoring, are likely to be instructive. As a pervasive complication associated with clinically relevant outcomes, postoperative delirium is an area ripe for further research, with the potential to truly impact the way we care for hospitalized patients.

CONFLICT OF INTEREST STATEMENT

E.L.W., M.S.A, and S.K.I. have no conflicts of interest to disclose.

REFERENCES

1. Steiner LA. Postoperative delirium. Part 1: pathophysiology and risk factors. *Eur J Anaesthesiol.* 2011;28:628–636.
2. Radtke FM, Franck M, Lorenz M, et al. Remifentanil reduces the incidence of post-operative delirium. *J Int Med Res.* 2010;38:1225–1232.

3. Pandharipande P, Cotton BA, Shintani A, et al. Prevalence and risk factors for development of delirium in surgical and trauma intensive care unit patients. *J Trauma*. 2008;65:34–41.

4. Kazmierski J, Kowman M, Banach M, et al. Incidence and predictors of delirium after cardiac surgery: results from the IPDACS Study. *J Psychosom Res*. 2010;69:179–185.

5. Rudolph JL, Inouye SK, Jones RN, et al. Delirium: an independent predictor of functional decline after cardiac surgery. *J Am Geriatr Soc*. 2010;58:643–649.

6. Rudolph JL, Jones RN, Levkoff SE, et al. Derivation and validation of a preoperative prediction rule for delirium after cardiac surgery. *Circulation*. 2009;119:229–236.

7. Fisher BW, Flowerdew G. A simple model for predicting postoperative delirium in older patients undergoing elective orthopedic surgery. *J Am Geriatr Soc*. 1995;43:175–178.

8. Marcantonio ER, Flacker JM, Michaels M, Resnick NM. Delirium is independently associated with poor functional recovery after hip fracture. *J Am Geriatr Soc*. 2000;48:618–624.

9. Lee KH, Ha YC, Lee YK, Kang H, Koo KH. Frequency, risk factors, and prognosis of prolonged delirium in elderly patients after hip fracture surgery. *Clin Orthop Relat Res*. 2011;469:2612–2620.

10. Rudolph JL, Marcantonio ER. Review articles: postoperative delirium: acute change with long-term implications. *Anesth Analg*. 2011;112:1202–1211.

11. Gottesman RF, Grega MA, Bailey MM, et al. Delirium after coronary artery bypass graft surgery and late mortality. *Ann Neurol*. 2010;67:338–344.

12. Koster S, Hensens AG, Schuurmans MJ, van der Palen J. Consequences of delirium after cardiac operations. *Ann Thorac Surg*. 2012;93:705–711.

13. Kat MG, Vreeswijk R, de Jonghe JF, et al. Long-term cognitive outcome of delirium in elderly hip surgery patients. A prospective matched controlled study over two and a half years. *Dement Geriatr Cogn Disord*. 2008;26:1–8.

14. Brouquet A, Cudennec T, Benoist S, et al. Impaired mobility, ASA status and administration of tramadol are risk factors for postoperative delirium in patients aged 75 years or more after major abdominal surgery. *Ann Surg*. 2010;251:759–765.

15. Franco K, Litaker D, Locala J, Bronson D. The cost of delirium in the surgical patient. *Psychosomatics*. 2001;42:68–73.

16. Bickel H, Gradinger R, Kochs E, Forstl H. High risk of cognitive and functional decline after postoperative delirium. A three-year prospective study. *Dement Geriatr Cogn Disord*. 2008;26:26–31.

17. Leslie DL, Marcantonio ER, Zhang Y, Leo-Summers L, Inouye SK. One-year health care costs associated with delirium in the elderly population. *Arch Intern Med*. 2008;168:27–32.

18. Koster S, Hensens AG, Schuurmans MJ, van der Palen J. Risk factors of delirium after cardiac surgery: a systematic review. *Eur J Cardiovasc Nurs*. 2011;10:197–204.

19. Jones RN, Fong TG, Metzger E, et al. Aging, brain disease, and reserve: implications for delirium. *Am J Geriatr Psychiatry*. 2010;18:117–127.

20. Patti R, Saitta M, Cusumano G, Termine G, Di Vita G. Risk factors for postoperative delirium after colorectal surgery for carcinoma. *Eur J Oncol Nurs*. 2011;15:519–523.

21. Radtke FM, Franck M, MacGuill M, et al. Duration of fluid fasting and choice of analgesic are modifiable factors for early postoperative delirium. *Eur J Anaesthesiol*. 2010;27(5):411–416.

22. Morimoto Y, Yoshimura M, Utada K, Setoyama K, Matsumoto M, Sakabe T. Prediction of postoperative delirium after abdominal surgery in the elderly. *J Anesth*. 2009;23:51–56.

23. Schoen J, Meyerose J, Paarmann H, Heringlake M, Hueppe M, Berger KU. Preoperative regional cerebral oxygen saturation is a predictor of postoperative delirium in on-pump cardiac surgery patients: a prospective observational trial. *Crit Care*. 2011;15:R218.

24. Siepe M, Pfeiffer T, Gieringer A, et al. Increased systemic perfusion pressure during cardiopulmonary bypass is associated with less early postoperative cognitive dysfunction and delirium. *Eur J Cardiothorac Surg*. 2011;40:200–207.

25. Inouye SK, Bogardus ST, Jr., Charpentier PA, et al. A multicomponent intervention to prevent delirium in hospitalized older patients. *N Engl J Med*. 1999;340:669–676.

26. Rubin FH, Neal K, Fenlon K, Hassan S, Inouye SK. Sustainability and scalability of the hospital elder life program at a community hospital. *J Am Geriatr Soc*. 2011;59:359–365.

27. Rubin FH, Williams JT, Lescisin DA, Mook WJ, Hassan S, Inouye SK. Replicating the Hospital Elder Life Program in a community hospital and demonstrating effectiveness using quality improvement methodology. *J Am Geriatr Soc*. 2006;54:969–974.

28. Inouye SK, Bogardus ST, Jr., Baker DI, Leo-Summers L, Cooney LM, Jr. The Hospital Elder Life Program: a model of care to prevent cognitive and functional decline in older hospitalized patients. Hospital Elder Life Program. *J Am Geriatr Soc*. 2000;48:1697–1706.

29. Caplan GA, Harper EL. Recruitment of volunteers to improve vitality in the elderly: the REVIVE study. *Intern Med J*. 2007;37:95–100.

30. Leslie DL, Zhang Y, Bogardus ST, Holford TR, Leo-Summers LS, Inouye SK. Consequences of preventing delirium in hospitalized older adults on nursing home costs. *J Am Geriatr Soc*. 2005;53:405–409.

31. Rizzo JA, Bogardus ST, Jr., Leo-Summers L, Williams CS, Acampora D, Inouye SK. Multicomponent targeted intervention to prevent delirium in hospitalized older patients: what is the economic value? *Med Care*. 2001;39:740–752.

32. Chen CC, Lin MT, Tien YW, Yen CJ, Huang GH, Inouye SK. Modified hospital elder life program: effects on abdominal surgery patients. *J Am Coll Surg*. 2011;213:245–252.

33. Marcantonio ER, Flacker JM, Wright RJ, Resnick NM. Reducing delirium after hip fracture: a randomized trial. *J Am Geriatr Soc*. 2001;49:516–522.

34. Sanders RD. Hypothesis for the pathophysiology of delirium: role of baseline brain network connectivity and changes in inhibitory tone. *Med Hypotheses*. 2011;77:140–143.

35. Mason SE, Noel-Storr A, Ritchie CW. The impact of general and regional anesthesia on the incidence of post-operative cognitive dysfunction and post-operative delirium: a systematic review with meta-analysis. *J Alzheimers Dis*. 2010;22 Suppl 3:67–79.

36. Sieber FE, Zakriya KJ, Gottschalk A, et al. Sedation depth during spinal anesthesia and the development of postoperative delirium in elderly patients undergoing hip fracture repair. *Mayo Clin Proc*. 2010;85:18–26.

37. Kalisvaart KJ, de Jonghe JF, Bogaards MJ, et al. Haloperidol prophylaxis for elderly hip-surgery patients at risk for delirium: a randomized placebo-controlled study. *J Am Geriatr Soc*. 2005;53:1658–1666.

38. Wang W, Li HL, Wang DX, et al. Haloperidol prophylaxis decreases delirium incidence in elderly patients after noncardiac surgery: a randomized controlled trial. *Crit Care Med*. 2012;40:731–739.

39. National Institute for Health and Clinical Excellence. Delirium: diagnosis, prevention, and management (clinical guideline 103). 2010. http://www.nice.org.uk/nicemedia/live/13060/49909/49909.pdf. Accessed November 11, 2012.

40. Neufeld KJ, Hayat MJ, Coughlin JM, et al. Evaluation of two intensive care delirium screening tools for non-critically ill hospitalized patients. *Psychosomatics*. 2011;52:133–140.

41. van Eijk MM, van den Boogaard M, van Marum RJ, et al. Routine use of the confusion assessment method for the intensive care unit: a multicenter study. *Am J Respir Crit Care Med*. 2011;184:340–344.

42. Greer N, Rossom R, Anderson P, et al. Delirium: screening, prevention, and diagnosis—a systematic review of the evidence. VA-ESP Project #09–009 2011. http:www.hsrd.research.va.gov/publications/esp/delirium.pdf.

3.

POSTOPERATIVE COGNITIVE TRAJECTORY

Robert D. Sanders, Mervyn Maze, Alex S. Evers, and Michael S. Avidan

INTRODUCTION TO THE CLINICAL PROBLEM

For the last 60 years there has been a strong perception that some elderly patients experience persistent cognitive decline that is directly attributable to a surgical event, to receiving general anesthesia, or to a combination of insults involving both surgery and general anesthesia.[1] For certain surgeries, notably cardiac surgery and major orthopedic surgery, persistent postoperative cognitive decline (POCD) has been thought to affect up to 50% of patients.[2,3] Based on limited clinical data[4] as well as laboratory experimentation,[5–9] it has been hypothesized that surgery and anesthesia could either accelerate the onset of dementia or even cause dementia, and that POCD could be a harbinger of subsequent dementia.[8] If these concerns regarding persistent POCD were proven to be true, then we would have a major public health problem, and it would be necessary for older patients to factor persistent POCD into their decision making regarding the potential pros and cons of undergoing a surgical procedure.

Postoperative delirium is recognized to be a common and clinically important complication,[10–13] covered in Chapter 2. It is also generally appreciated that cognition is frequently impaired for several weeks following surgery,[10,14,15] analogous to the cognitive impairment that occurs with acute medical illnesses. Furthermore, there is increasing evidence to suggest that pain and inflammation carry a cognitive burden;[16,17] people who have chronic inflammatory states or unremitting pain could suffer from accelerated cognitive decline.[18–21] However, research in the last decade has challenged established views on POCD, especially regarding how persistent the cognitive decline really is.[10,22,23] Indeed, some studies suggest that when surgery successfully removes the cause of the preoperative disability, the quality of life, functional status, and cognition might all improve.[17,24–27]

Absent a clear consensus about the definition, time course, and clinical impact of POCD, it is not surprising that the literature is permeated with data from studies that lack prospective designs, appropriate nonsurgical control groups, detection of pre-existing cognitive impairment, information on preoperative cognitive trajectory, long-term follow-up, and appropriate statistical analyses. In this chapter, we shall sift through the evidence and address whether there is a vulnerable subgroup of patients who might be afflicted by long-lasting cognitive decline and, conversely, whether some patients may exhibit a postoperative cognitive improvement (POCI). From the outset it is necessary to qualify, especially for readers unfamiliar with the evidence and the controversies in this field, that the published literature can be interpreted in various ways; currently there is a range of views surrounding the clinical relevance of persistent POCD. In the last few years, several clinical review articles have been published on POCD and postoperative dementia.[23,28–37] While consensus on many issues is emerging, some of the emphases and nuances expressed in scientific reviews differ from the viewpoints we express in this chapter. Reading some of these pertinent review articles might help to enrich perspectives on this controversial topic.

INCIDENCE, PREVALENCE, AND OUTCOMES

The incidence of POCD is difficult to determine, for several reasons. First, elderly people decline cognitively, and over time a substantial number of older people develop dementia. The prevalence of dementia in people over the age of 60 is estimated to be >5%.[38,39] The prevalence of Alzheimer's disease specifically almost doubles every 5 years after age 65, leading to a prevalence of >25% in those over the age of 90.[39,40] Therefore, any study that follows older people longitudinally will observe cognitive decline and incident dementia. If older people are followed after a surgical event without an appropriate control group, cognitive decline and incident dementia might be incorrectly attributed to the surgery.[41] Also, many older patients undergoing surgical procedures have comorbidities, such as vascular disease, that are themselves associated with cognitive decline and dementia.[23,40,41] Again, this could lead to an incorrect attribution of cognitive decline or incident dementia to a surgical event, rather than to other risk factors.[23,41]

The third reason it is difficult to determine the incidence of POCD is that it is hard to assess patients' postoperative cognitive trajectories if preoperative cognitive trajectories have not been established. There is compelling evidence that patients who have declining trajectories before surgery or those who have mild cognitive impairment or early dementia prior to surgery are more likely to decline cognitively after surgery.[10,42] In addition, there is no consensus definition for POCD, and the quoted incidence varies widely (e.g., from 5% to 50%) depending on the arbitrary diagnostic criteria that have been used.[3,22] For example, a very liberal criterion that has been used is a standard deviation decline in any of several administered cognitive tests, regardless of whether or not patients improve on any of the other cognitive tests. With such a permissive definition, it is likely that POCD would be diagnosed purely by chance in about a third of all patients.[43]

Finally, with repeat cognitive testing, there is a learning effect, and studies have tried to correct for learning, often based on measured learning in a reference group. However, this assumes that learning in surgical patients is relatively uniform and that the learning effect is as marked among those who are undergoing a surgical procedure as it is in the typically nonsurgical reference group. This assumption is unlikely to be appropriate as patients who are distracted by the prospect of surgery are not likely to learn as efficiently as control subjects who are not confronting surgery. Therefore, correcting for learning based on a nonsurgical control group could lead to an overestimate of the extent or incidence of POCD. This limitation was made salient in a study by Evered et al.,[44] which enrolled four cohorts: patients undergoing cardiac surgery, patients undergoing orthopedic surgery, a control group undergoing coronary angiography, and a second control group not undergoing any procedure. Using the results in the nonprocedural control group to correct for learning, the investigators found that at 3 months the cohort that underwent coronary angiography (i.e., no surgery and no general anesthesia) had the highest incidence of cognitive decline. These results demonstrate that correcting for learning in a surgical (or procedural) group according to learning in a nonsurgical control group could lead to an artificial diagnosis of POCD. Alternative statistical approaches, such as mixed effects models, have been used in studies of POCD and are probably more robust than methods that rely on correction for learning based on a nonprocedural control group[23,42,45] (Figures 3.1a and 3.1b).

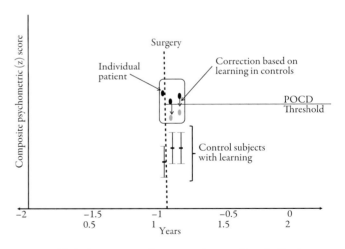

Figure 3.1A Typical assessment of postoperative cognitive decline in outcomes studies. In many studies, patients undergo baseline cognitive assessment prior to surgery and follow-up assessments at 1 to 4 weeks postoperatively and again at 3 months postoperatively. In this figure, a representative patient declines slightly on some of the cognitive tests and in a composite cognitive score at the two postoperative intervals. The patient's scores at these time points are adjusted down on the basis of mean divided by standard deviation of improvement (learning) in a matched nonsurgical control group. Following this correction, the patient crosses an arbitrary statistical threshold (e.g., decline by >2 standard deviations in a composite cognitive score) and is diagnosed with postoperative cognitive decline (POCD).

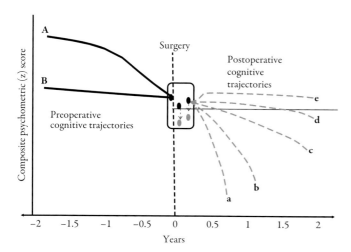

Figure 3.1B Preoperative and postoperative cognitive trajectories. In this figure, possible preoperative and postoperative cognitive trajectories are shown for the patient in Figure 3.1A. Curve **A** is representative of a patient who is experiencing cognitive decline preoperatively, while curve **B** represents a patient with relatively stable preoperative cognition. If Patient **A** were to have curve **b** as a postoperative trajectory, that would be an extension of the preoperative trend. Curve **a** would be an acceleration of cognitive decline, and curve **c** would be deceleration in cognitive decline, or cognitive improvement, compared with the expected or extrapolated trajectory. Without knowledge of this patient's preoperative trajectory, all three curves (**a**, **b**, **c**) would reasonably be interpreted as postoperative cognitive decline. In relation to patient **B**'s preoperative cognitive trajectory, curve **c** shows postoperative cognitive decline, curve **d** represents a continuation of the preoperative course, and curve **e** suggest postoperative cognitive improvement. Interestingly, curve **c** represents relative cognitive improvement for patient **A** and relative cognitive decline for patient **B**.

EARLY POCD

In the first few weeks to months following surgery, many patients are debilitated, in pain, and unable to function in daily life as they did before surgery. Unsurprisingly, during this period, POCD and general decrements of quality-of-life measures are common. POCD in the early postoperative period is clinically relevant because of its probable adverse impact on recovery of function and because in two studies an association has been found between early POCD and intermediate-term (1–2 years) postoperative mortality.[46,47] Furthermore, early POCD has been found to be a risk factor for early departure from the workforce.[47]

The International Study of POCD (ISPOCD), a research consortium founded in 1994 (http://www.sps.ele.tue.nl/ispocd/sub0/main.html), has made major contributions to the study of POCD. In a seminal study published in the *Lancet*, ISPOCD investigators found that 10% of older patients undergoing major noncardiac surgery met the ISPOCD diagnostic criteria for POCD at 3 months postoperatively.[14] In order to meet the diagnosis of POCD, patients had to decline by >2 standard deviations on at least

two out of seven cognitive tests, or by >2 standard deviations in a composite cognitive score. Subsequent to this landmark publication, other studies, using a similar approach, have corroborated these findings of POCD at 3 months.[15,48] Importantly, these studies have generally corrected for the learning effect using the so-called reliable change index, a correction factor based on the average divided by the standard deviation of learning in a nonsurgical control group.[49,50] Also, these studies have focused on evidence of decline and have tended to view evidence of cognitive improvement as statistical artifact.

PERSISTENT POCD

Two influential studies have reported that almost half of cardiac and noncardiac surgical patients have persistent POCD.[2,3] In the case of cardiac surgery patients, this cognitive decline was reported 5 years after surgery[2] and for the noncardiac surgical patients the decline was measured at 1 year.[3] Both of these studies diagnosed cognitive decline using the permissive definition of >1 standard deviation decline in any cognitive domain. Neither study reported cognitive improvement according to the reciprocal diagnostic criterion. Furthermore, these studies did not include an appropriate, matched nonsurgical control group, making it impossible to determine the extent to which cognitive decline, if indeed present, was attributable to the surgical event. Despite their methodological weaknesses, these studies have reinforced the pervasive view among clinicians and members of the public alike that lasting cognitive decline, affecting quality of life and function, is common after surgery.

A review of cardiac and noncardiac surgical studies reported that when studies included appropriate nonsurgical control groups,[22,41,42,45,51–54] persistent POCD was generally not found.[29] A study by Ballard et al. from the United Kingdom yielded provocative results.[55] This study enrolled 192 patients undergoing abdominal and orthopedic surgery, as well as an age-matched control group (n = 138). Surprisingly, after correcting for learning in the control group, the investigators found that even with use of more stringent POCD diagnostic criteria (>2 SD decline in >2 tests or in a composite score), 11.2% of surgical patients had POCD at 1 year postoperatively compared with cognitive decline in 3.8% of controls ($p = 0.02$). One important question in relation to these results is whether the control group was appropriately matched with the surgical patients in terms of baseline cognition, comorbidities, and risk factors for cognitive decline. Nevertheless, these data suggest that there might be some patients who are at risk for persistent POCD.

ALZHEIMER'S DISEASE AND OTHER DEMENTIAS

Several in vitro and animal experiments have suggested that general anesthetic agents, especially isoflurane, might initiate or accelerate pathologic processes (e.g., generation of β-amyloid of phosphorylated tau protein in the brain) that have been associated with the pathogenesis of Alzheimer's disease.[5,9,56–59] One observational clinical study in cardiac surgery patients has found a potential link between heart surgery and subsequent incident dementia.[4] Other studies have generally not found a suggestion of a causal link between surgery and subsequent dementia.[29] It has yet to be determined in humans whether a single (uncomplicated) surgery or exposure to general anesthesia could increase the risk of subsequent incident dementia.

RISK FACTORS

Given the subtle nature of POCD and the variability in diagnostic criteria, it is not surprising that there is a lack of robust data on the risk factors for POCD. This is compounded by difficulties in statistical adjustment for all potential risk factors to get a measure of the importance of the effect.

AGE

A relatively consistent finding is the relationship of increasing age with increased risk of POCD at 1 week and at 3 months.[15,46,60] It has been suggested that this is attributable to a fall in "cognitive reserve." However, it is unclear to what extent comorbidities confound the impact of age. While some studies have considered preoperative cognition, vascular risk factors, or perioperative variables, a more holistic approach is required to identify accurately vulnerable subgroups of patients who may develop POCD.

PREOPERATIVE COGNITION

While higher education status is suggested to protect against cognitive decline at 1 week,[14] a major risk factor for POCD is a preoperative cognitive impairment and decline.[10,42] However, the question of whether the cognitive trajectory changes postoperatively is incompletely addressed; evidence based on patients with mild cognitive impairment who have undergone surgery is conflicting in this regard.[42,61] An innovative study by Kline et al. examined data from the Alzheimer Disease Neuroimaging Initiative (ADNI), including participants who underwent surgical procedures (n = 41) and propensity-matched control participants who did not undergo surgery (n = 123).[62] The investigators found that patients who had mild cognitive impairment or early dementia prior to surgery experienced POCD within the first few months postoperatively.[62] They also found that on structural magnetic resonance imaging, there was evidence of postoperative atrophy in the cortex and hippocampus in the participants who underwent surgery.[62] Interestingly, both the cognitive decline and the brain atrophy were subsequently reversed in many subjects,[62] pointing to neuroplasticity throughout life and the potential for both cognitive decline and improvement following surgery.

CARDIOPULMONARY BYPASS

To this day there remains a strong perception that heart surgery, especially with cardiopulmonary bypass, is associated with a high risk of POCD. This concern was so compelling that off-pump cardiac surgery was developed, largely in attempt to prevent cardiopulmonary bypass-associated cognitive decline. However, large clinical trials that have randomized patients to heart surgery with or without cardiopulmonary bypass have found no difference in postoperative cognitive trajectories between groups. While cognitive decline might occur following cardiac surgery, it is difficult to ascertain whether the decline is attributable to the cardiac surgery or whether the decline is related to comorbidites, such as vascular disease. For example, studies from Johns Hopkins have examined patients who have undergone cardiac surgery and have compared them with nonsurgical control patients both with and without vascular disease.[45,54] Interestingly, these studies have shown that the rate of cognitive decline over years was no different between those with vascular disease who underwent heart surgery and those with coronary vascular disease who were nonsurgically treated. The heart-healthy control group did not decline cognitively at the same rate. The investigators suggested that generalized vascular disease might be a potent risk factor for cognitive decline rather than coronary surgery, which had previously been implicated. In an article distilling the evidence, Selnes et al. commented, "it is now increasingly apparent that the incidence of both short- and long-term cognitive decline after CABG (coronary artery bypass grafting) has been greatly overestimated, owing to the lack of a uniform definition of what constitutes cognitive decline, the use of inappropriate statistical methods, and a lack of control groups."[23]

In the last 15 years, several studies have randomized patients with coronary artery disease to receive either surgery or percutaneous coronary intervention.[24,26,63] These trials have provided an important opportunity to judge whether cardiac surgery and general anesthesia are really potent independent agents of cognitive decline and decrements in quality of life. The trials have not demonstrated that patients randomized to surgery had worse cognitive outcomes, and generally, quality of life was improved whether patients underwent surgical treatment or percutaneous coronary intervention.[26] A recent meta-analysis, which included 28 studies with 2,043 patients who underwent CABG surgery,[64] corroborated the emerging evidence suggesting that persistent cognitive decline is probably not as common as previously reported following heart surgery. Indeed, contrary to expectations, this meta-analysis found that, on aggregate, there was improvement in overall cognitive function in the first year following CABG surgery.[64]

VASCULAR RISK FACTORS

Vascular risk factors, such as hypertension, smoking and atherosclerosis, are strongly associated with cognitive decline in the general population[40,65] and with postoperative delirium.[66] Indeed, patients who underwent either surgical coronary artery bypass grafting or percutaneous coronary intervention for treatment of their cardiac condition experienced a similar degree of cognitive decline over time.[67] Therefore, the cognitive decline was probably attributable to the progression of vascular disease rather than the studied interventions. Interestingly, there is evidence that antihypertensive interventions might reduce the incidence or slow progression of vascular dementia.[65,68]

INTRAOPERATIVE TECHNIQUES

An association between general anesthesia and POCD and Alzheimer's disease has also been debated, though the weight of evidence suggests no firm association. Authors of many studies comparing regional and general anesthesia during surgery have looked at cognitive outcomes, but synthesis of the data showed no association.[69,70] A meta-analysis of 21 trials showed that general anesthesia was marginally, but nonsignificantly, associated with POCD (odds ratio of 1.34; 95% confidence interval, 0.93 to 1.95).[33] If, despite the current negative evidence, general anesthesia does independently contribute to POCD, it is likely that its contribution is minor.

The ISPOCD group tested the association of hypoxia or hypotension with POCD at 1 week and 3 months but were unable to find an association. Therefore, while it seems plausible that hypotension contributes to POCD as it might contribute to perioperative mortality,[71] evidence is lacking for a firm contribution. However, loss of cerebral autoregulation in patients with vascular risk factors, such as hypertension, may increase the vulnerability of these patients to POCD as it is thought to for delirium.[72] A small randomized, controlled study suggested that guiding anesthetic management with a processed electroencephalogram monitor and cerebral oximetry might be associated with decreased incidence of POCD 1 year postoperatively.[55] The investigators suggested that avoiding unnecessarily deep anesthesia and maintaining adequate cerebral oxygen supply could be important approaches to protecting the brain from subtle damage during surgery. These intriguing results are hypothesis generating and should be tested in larger studies.

POSTOPERATIVE DELIRIUM

Although delirium is addressed in Chapter 2, it is important to emphasize here that delirium, an acute and fluctuating brain disorder, occurs in 10% to 70% of patients older than 65 undergoing major surgical procedures.[73] The association between delirium and POCD is unclear, and findings have conflicted in different studies. Some studies have found that postoperative delirium predicts early POCD lasting weeks to months,[10,74,75] while others have not found an association.[76,77] Although POCD associated with postoperative delirium has generally been shown to resolve, research has shown that patients who experience postoperative delirium are at markedly increased risk for subsequent cognitive decline, incident dementia, and severe dependency in activities of daily living measured 2 to 3 years after surgery.[78,79] A study by Saczynski et al. showed that patients who had delirium after heart surgery had marked early postoperative POCD, which in some patients appeared to persist for up to 6 months.[10] Somewhat surprisingly, patients in this study with postoperative delirium and early POCD appeared to return to baseline cognition within the first postoperative year.[10] It is important to qualify that cognition in this study was tracked with the Mini Mental Status Test, which is intended as a screening test for dementia and is not regarded as a valid psychometric instrument for tracking cognition.

One possible explanation for the apparently discrepant findings is that patients who have brain pathology but have not yet manifested clinical evidence of dementia might be more likely to develop postoperative delirium. If this were true, postoperative delirium could be a marker of brain pathology, decreased cognitive reserve, and a harbinger of future cognitive decline and dementia. Conceptually, major surgery and general anesthesia could be thought of a stress test for the brain, and postoperative delirium could be a positive stress test, revealing brain vulnerability.

OTHER POSTOPERATIVE COMPLICATIONS

The ISPOCD also looked at the effect of respiratory and infectious complications on risk of POCD, finding an association at 1 week but not 3 months.[14] These complications may have been associated with delirium or may have exerted an independent effect on short-term cognition. Through a similar mechanism to increasing delirium, the accompanying inflammation may have increased the risk of POCD.

GENETIC FACTORS

It has been hypothesized that genetic risk factors for POCD would probably overlap with those for neurodegenerative disorders, such as Alzheimer's disease. The ε4 allele of the apolipoprotein E gene is a known risk factor for Alzheimer's disease, poor outcome after cerebral injury, and accelerated cognitive decline with normal aging.[80] No association has been demonstrated between the apolipoprotein E genotype and POCD.[3,74,80] It remains possible that there are people with a genetic predisposition to developing POCD. A major challenge is that because there are no consensus diagnostic criteria for POCD, detecting an association between candidate genotypes and the phenotype (i.e., POCD) is likely to be problematic.[81] Interestingly, genetic factors, such as variants in the amyloid-β precursor protein gene, have also been found that are protective against Alzheimer's disease and general cognitive decline in the elderly.[82] Such factors might also confer protection against POCD.

INFLAMMATION

That the trauma of surgery is capable of engaging the innate immune system and eliciting an inflammatory response has been known for decades. However, recently reported preclinical data have revealed that the brain is also affected by peripheral surgery through a series of steps that culminate in the recruitment of activated monocytes/macrophages into the hippocampus where they release proinflammatory cytokines capable of disrupting hippocampal long-term potentiation (LTP), the neurobiologic correlate of learning and memory formation.[83,84] This sequence of events gives rise to "sickness behavior" consisting of lethargy, anorexia, loss of sexual interest, fever, and cognitive dysfunction, a constellation of symptoms that may serve to nullify the need or desire for the injured organism to leave its "cave;"

thus, inflammation-induced wound healing can proceed without exposing the animal to further damage.

Data have begun to accumulate indicating that inflammation itself activates a resolving mechanism that limits further engagement of the innate immune response.[85] A vagally mediated neural reflex eventually activates the α_7 nicotinic acetylcholine receptor on the monocyte at its terminus in the spleen; this limits further synthesis of proinflammatory cytokines by inhibiting the action of the transcription factor NF-κB.[85] When this vagal reflex is disrupted, neuroinflammation and cognitive decline persist. Perioperative drugs are capable of interfering with this vagal reflex; after benzodiazepines, drugs with anticholinergic activity (including meperidine and phenothiazines) are most likely to produce postoperative delirium.

Interestingly, the surgical patient with metabolic syndrome may be at increased risk of developing delirium and cognitive decline, possibly through dysfunctional cholinergic processes.[86] In a rat model of the metabolic syndrome, surgery exaggerated the transient acute state (postoperative day [POD] 7) and induced a prolonged cognitive decline (5 months). Preliminary data reveal a dysregulated cholinergic inflammation-resolving mechanism, although a causal link to cognitive decline is not yet established. However, surgical patients with longstanding chronic inflammatory conditions may also exhibit cognitive impairment. Thus it is conceivable that a surgical cure of the source of the inflammation may result in a postoperative improvement in cognitive function.

PREVENTIVE STRATEGIES AND TREATMENT

Current evidence suggests that POCD is generally a transient phenomenon, and patients whose surgery goes well, recover well. The promotion of successful surgery and active rehabilitation, as well as the avoidance of postoperative complications, such as wound infections and venous thromboses, are likely to decrease postoperative inflammation, which carries a cognitive burden. Patients who have complications of surgery and become critically ill could have a severe systemic inflammatory response syndrome and could develop multiorgan dysfunction, including the lungs, kidneys, heart, and brain. Fortunately, this is rare for elective surgery, although it might be much more common for patients on intensive care units with severe illness.

The most common persistent surgical complication, which might be germane to POCD, is persistent pain. Possibly through its association with inflammation, pain carries a cognitive burden, and cognition is likely to be impaired in chronic-pain sufferers. Some of the medications for chronic pain, such as opioids, could also hamper cognition and could contribute to persistent POCD. Therefore, multimodal perioperative strategies to prevent persistent pain might be helpful in preventing persistent POCD.

It has been shown that the brain retains neuroplastic potential throughout life; both cognitive improvement and cognitive decline are possible postoperative sequelae. As noted previously, several rigorous studies have suggested that quality of life, and perhaps even cognition, might be improved following cardiac surgery.[24,26] Studies that have combined neuroimaging, pain, and functional assessments have shown that when back surgery or hip replacement surgery is successful, cognition improves and gray matter increases in areas such as the dorsolateral prefrontal cortex, the anterior cingulate cortex, and the amygdala.[17,27] The possibility of postoperative cognitive improvement would be of tremendous relevance and comfort to surgical patients and could be an important objective for perioperative clinicians. Promoting physical and cerebral fitness through exercise programs and structured brain-training initiatives are interventions that theoretically could enhance cognition. The most important interventions to promote postoperative cognitive health are probably to promote rehabilitation, prevent medical complications of surgery, and be proactive in treating postoperative pain.

CURRENT GUIDELINES AND RECOMMENDATIONS

At present it would be premature to issue guidelines on POCD. The lack of robust data indicating that this is a long-term problem or on risk factors to help identify vulnerable subgroups makes counseling the patient difficult. Patients should not be dissuaded from having surgery because of fears over a change in cognition. It also seems sensible to avoid benzodiazepines in patients at risk of delirium and early POCD, to reduce the burden of these conditions. In the meantime, we must continue to pursue clinical and preclinical studies to quantify the extent of this problem, especially to identify any vulnerable subgroup of patients, and to understand the pathogenesis of POCD and delirium.

CONCLUSION

Whether or not persistent POCD exists as a clinically important medical problem remains unclear. There is mounting evidence that some patients do decline cognitively following surgery. The most common reason is probably that these patients were already declining before surgery. However, there are additional patients who appear to experience de novo or accelerated cognitive decline. These patients might have postoperative medical complications; they might suffer from marked pain and inflammation; their surgery might be associated with major tissue trauma or technical problems; they might be susceptible to anesthetic induced neurotoxicity; or their surgery might exacerbate pre-existing cognitive decline. On the other hand, it is also probable that there are some patients who improve cognitively after surgery. These patients might be those whose surgery improves function, treats a medical condition, or ultimately decreases pain and inflammation. We echo the sentiment expressed by Selnes et al.: "Most patients in whom new cognitive symptoms develop during the immediate postoperative period can be reassured that these symptoms generally resolve within 1 to 3 months."[23] Furthermore, if surgery goes well, resulting in decreased pain and inflammation and increased functionality, postoperative improvements in quality of life and cognition are realistic and desirable outcomes.

CONFLICT OF INTEREST STATEMENT

R.S. has acted as a consultant for Air Liquide, Paris, France, concerning the development of medical gases and has received speaker fees from Hospira, Chicago, USA, and Orion Pharmaceuticals, Turku, Finland. None of these companies had any involvement in this article.

M.M. is a co-inventor of a patent regarding xenon for neuroprotection.

A.S. E. serves on the Scientific Advisory Board of SAGE Therapeutics, Cambridge, Mass.

M.S.A. has no conflicts of interest to disclose.

REFERENCES

1. Bedford PD. Adverse cerebral effects of anaesthesia on old people. *Lancet*. 1955;269(6884):259–263.
2. Newman MF, Kirchner JL, Phillips-Bute B, et al. Longitudinal assessment of neurocognitive function after coronary-artery bypass surgery. *N Engl J Med*. 2001;344(6):395–402.
3. McDonagh DL, Mathew JP, White WD, et al. Cognitive function after major noncardiac surgery, apolipoprotein E4 genotype, and biomarkers of brain injury. *Anesthesiology*. 2010;112(4):852–859.
4. Lee TA, Wolozin B, Weiss KB, Bednar MM. Assessment of the emergence of Alzheimer's disease following coronary artery bypass graft surgery or percutaneous transluminal coronary angioplasty. *J Alzheimers Dis*. 2005;7(4):319–324.

5. Eckenhoff RG, Johansson JS, Wei H, et al. Inhaled anesthetic enhancement of amyloid-beta oligomerization and cytotoxicity. *Anesthesiology*. 2004;101(3):703–709.

6. Liang G, Wang Q, Li Y, et al. A presenilin-1 mutation renders neurons vulnerable to isoflurane toxicity. *Anesth Analg*. 2008;106(2):492–500.

7. Wei H, Liang G, Yang H, et al. The common inhalational anesthetic isoflurane induces apoptosis via activation of inositol 1,4,5-trisphosphate receptors. *Anesthesiology*. 2008;108(2):251–260.

8. Baranov D, Bickler PE, Crosby GJ, et al. Consensus statement: First International Workshop on Anesthetics and Alzheimer's Disease. *Anesth Analg*. 2009;108(5):1627–1630.

9. Carnini A, Lear JD, Eckenhoff RG. Inhaled anesthetic modulation of amyloid beta(1-40) assembly and growth. *Curr Alzheimer Res*. 2007;4(3):233–241.

10. Saczynski JS, Marcantonio ER, Quach L, et al. Cognitive trajectories after postoperative delirium. *N Engl J Med*. 2012;367(1):30–39.

11. Leslie DL, Marcantonio ER, Zhang Y, Leo-Summers L, Inouye SK. One-year health care costs associated with delirium in the elderly population. *Arch Intern Med*. 2008;168(1):27–32.

12. Robinson TN, Raeburn CD, Tran ZV, Angles EM, Brenner LA, Moss M. Postoperative delirium in the elderly: risk factors and outcomes. *Ann Surg*. 2009;249(1):173–178.

13. Wacker P, Nunes PV, Cabrita H, Forlenza OV. Post-operative delirium is associated with poor cognitive outcome and dementia. *Dement Geriatr Cogn Disord*. 2006;21(4):221–227.

14. Moller JT, Cluitmans P, Rasmussen LS, et al. Long-term postoperative cognitive dysfunction in the elderly ISPOCD1 study. ISPOCD investigators. International Study of Post-Operative Cognitive Dysfunction. *Lancet*. 1998;351(9106):857–861.

15. Price CC, Garvan CW, Monk TG. Type and severity of cognitive decline in older adults after noncardiac surgery. *Anesthesiology*. 2008;108(1):8–17.

16. Terrando N, Monaco C, Ma D, Foxwell BM, Feldmann M, Maze M. Tumor necrosis factor-alpha triggers a cytokine cascade yielding postoperative cognitive decline. *Proc Natl Acad Sci U S A*. 2010;107(47):20518–20522.

17. Rodriguez-Raecke R, Niemeier A, Ihle K, Ruether W, May A. Brain gray matter decrease in chronic pain is the consequence and not the cause of pain. *J Neurosci*. 2009;29(44):13746–13750.

18. Holmes C, Cunningham C, Zotova E, et al. Systemic inflammation and disease progression in Alzheimer disease. *Neurology*. 2009;73(10):768–774.

19. Hu Z, Ou Y, Duan K, Jiang X. Inflammation: a bridge between postoperative cognitive dysfunction and Alzheimer's disease. *Med Hypotheses*. 2010;74(4):722–724.

20. Querfurth HW, LaFerla FM. Alzheimer's disease. *N Engl J Med*. 2010;362(4):329–344.

21. Fidalgo AR, Cibelli M, White JP, Nagy I, Maze M, Ma D. Systemic inflammation enhances surgery-induced cognitive dysfunction in mice. *Neurosci Lett*. 2011;498(1):63–66.

22. Abildstrom H, Rasmussen LS, Rentowl P, et al. Cognitive dysfunction 1-2 years after non-cardiac surgery in the elderly. ISPOCD group. International Study of Post-Operative Cognitive Dysfunction. *Acta Anaesthesiol Scand*. 2000;44(10):1246–1251.

23. Selnes OA, Gottesman RF, Grega MA, Baumgartner WA, Zeger SL, McKhann GM. Cognitive and neurologic outcomes after coronary-artery bypass surgery. *N Engl J Med*. 2012;366(3):250–257.

24. Wahrborg P, Booth JE, Clayton T, et al. Neuropsychological outcome after percutaneous coronary intervention or coronary artery bypass grafting: results from the Stent or Surgery (SoS) Trial. *Circulation*. 2004;110(22):3411–3417.

25. Van Dijk D, Jansen EW, Hijman R, Nierich AP, Diephuis JC, Moons KG, et al. Cognitive outcome after off-pump and on-pump coronary artery bypass graft surgery: a randomized trial. *JAMA*. 2002;287(11):1405–1412.

26. Cohen DJ, Van Hout B, Serruys PW, et al. Quality of life after PCI with drug-eluting stents or coronary-artery bypass surgery. *N Engl J Med*. 2011;364(11):1016–1026.

27. Seminowicz DA, Wideman TH, Naso L, et al. Effective treatment of chronic low back pain in humans reverses abnormal brain anatomy and function. *J Neurosci*. 2011;31(20):7540–7550.

28. Newman S, Stygall J, Hirani S, Shaefi S, Maze M. Postoperative cognitive dysfunction after noncardiac surgery: a systematic review. *Anesthesiology*. 2007;106(3):572–590.

29. Avidan MS, Evers AS. Review of clinical evidence for persistent cognitive decline or incident dementia attributable to surgery or general anesthesia. *J Alzheimer Dis*. 2011;24(2):201–216.

30. Deiner S, Silverstein JH. Postoperative delirium and cognitive dysfunction. *Br J Anaesth*. 2009;103(Suppl 1):i41–i46.

31. Rudolph JL, Schreiber KA, Culley DJ, et al. Measurement of post-operative cognitive dysfunction after cardiac surgery: a systematic review. *Acta Anaesthesiol Scand*. 2010;54(6):663–677.

32. Krenk L, Rasmussen LS, Kehlet H. New insights into the pathophysiology of postoperative cognitive dysfunction. *Acta Anaesthesiol Scand*. 2010;54(8):951–956.

33. Mason SE, Noel-Storr A, Ritchie CW. The impact of general and regional anesthesia on the incidence of post-operative cognitive dysfunction and post-operative delirium: a systematic review with meta-analysis. *J Alzheimers Dis*. 2010;22(Suppl 3):67–79.

34. Vanderweyde T, Bednar MM, Forman SA, Wolozin B. Iatrogenic risk factors for Alzheimer's disease: surgery and anesthesia. *J Alzheimers Dis*. 2010;22(Suppl 3):91–104.

35. Hudson AE, Hemmings HC, Jr. Are anaesthetics toxic to the brain? *Br J Anaesth*. 2011;107(1):30–37.

36. Monk TG, Price CC. Postoperative cognitive disorders. *Curr Opin Crit Care*. 2011;17(4):376–381.

37. Silbert B, Evered L, Scott DA. Cognitive decline in the elderly: is anaesthesia implicated? *Best Pract Res Clin Anaesthesiol*. 2011;25(3):379–393.

38. Ferri CP, Prince M, Brayne C, et al. Global prevalence of dementia: a Delphi consensus study. *Lancet*. 2005;366(9503):2112–2117.

39. 2012 Alzheimer's disease facts and figures. *Alzheimers Dement*. 2012;8(2):131–168.

40. Qiu C, Kivipelto M, von Strauss E. Epidemiology of Alzheimer's disease: occurrence, determinants, and strategies toward intervention. *Dialogues Clin Neurosci*. 2009;11(2):111–128.

41. van Dijk D, Moons KG, Nathoe HM, et al. Cognitive outcomes five years after not undergoing coronary artery bypass graft surgery. *Ann Thorac Surg*. 2008;85(1):60–64.

42. Avidan MS, Searleman AC, Storandt M, et al. Long-term cognitive decline in older subjects was not attributable to noncardiac surgery or major illness. *Anesthesiology*. 2009;111(5):964–970.

43. Keizer AM, Hijman R, Kalkman CJ, Kahn RS, van Dijk D. The incidence of cognitive decline after (not) undergoing coronary artery bypass grafting: the impact of a controlled definition. *Acta Anaesthesiol Scand*. 2005;49(9):1232–1235.

44. Evered L, Scott DA, Silbert B, Maruff P. Postoperative cognitive dysfunction is independent of type of surgery and anesthetic. *Anesth Analg*. 2011;112(5):1179–1185.

45. Selnes OA, Grega MA, Bailey MM, et al. Cognition 6 years after surgical or medical therapy for coronary artery disease. *Ann Neurol*. 2008;63(5):581–590.

46. Monk TG, Weldon BC, Garvan CW, et al. Predictors of cognitive dysfunction after major noncardiac surgery. *Anesthesiology*. 2008;108(1):18–30.

47. Steinmetz J, Christensen KB, Lund T, Lohse N, Rasmussen LS. Long-term consequences of postoperative cognitive dysfunction. *Anesthesiology*. 2009;110(3):548–555.

48. Johnson T, Monk T, Rasmussen LS, et al. Postoperative cognitive dysfunction in middle-aged patients. *Anesthesiology*. 2002;96(6):1351–1357.

49. Lewis MS, Maruff P, Silbert BS, Evered LA, Scott DA. The influence of different error estimates in the detection of post-operative cognitive dysfunction using reliable change indices with correction for practice effects. *Arch Clin Neuropsychol.* 2006;21(5):421–427.

50. Lewis MS, Maruff P, Silbert BS, Evered LA, Scott DA. The sensitivity and specificity of three common statistical rules for the classification of post-operative cognitive dysfunction following coronary artery bypass graft surgery. *Acta Anaesthesiol Scand.* 2006;50(1):50–57.

51. Gilberstadt H, Aberwald R, Crosbie S, Schuell H, Jimenez E. Effect of surgery on psychological and social functioning in elderly patients. *Arch Intern Med.* 1968;122(2):109–115.

52. Goldstein MZ, Fogel BS, Young BL. Effect of elective surgery under general anesthesia on mental status variables in elderly women and men: 10-month follow-up. *Int Psychogeriatrics/IPA.* 1996;8(1):135–149.

53. Ancelin ML, de Roquefeuil G, Scali J, et al. Long-term post-operative cognitive decline in the elderly: the effects of anesthesia type, apolipoprotein e genotype, and clinical antecedents. *J Alzheimers Dis.* 2010;22:105–113.

54. Selnes OA, Grega MA, Bailey MM, et al. Neurocognitive outcomes 3 years after coronary artery bypass graft surgery: a controlled study. *Ann Thorac Surg.* 2007;84(6):1885–1896.

55. Ballard C, Jones E, Gauge N, et al. Optimised anaesthesia to reduce post-operative cognitive decline (POCD) in older patients undergoing elective surgery, a randomised controlled trial. *PLoS One.* 2012;7(6):e37410.

56. Mandal PK, Pettegrew JW, McKeag DW, Mandal R. Alzheimer's disease: halothane induces Abeta peptide to oligomeric form—solution NMR studies. *Neurochem Res.* 2006;31(7):883–890.

57. Palotas M, Palotas A, Bjelik A, et al. Effect of general anesthetics on amyloid precursor protein and mRNA levels in the rat brain. *Neurochem Res.* 2005;30(8):1021–1026.

58. Planel E, Richter KE, Nolan CE, et al. Anesthesia leads to tau hyperphosphorylation through inhibition of phosphatase activity by hypothermia. *J Neurosci.* 2007;27(12):3090–3097.

59. Xie Z, Culley DJ, Dong Y, et al. The common inhalation anesthetic isoflurane induces caspase activation and increases amyloid beta-protein level in vivo. *Ann Neurol.* 2008;64(6):618–627.

60. Rasmussen LS, Steentoft A, Rasmussen H, Kristensen PA, Moller JT. Benzodiazepines and postoperative cognitive dysfunction in the elderly. ISPOCD Group. International Study of Postoperative Cognitive Dysfunction. *Br J Anaesth.* 1999;83(4):585–589.

61. Bekker A, Lee C, de Santi S, et al. Does mild cognitive impairment increase the risk of developing postoperative cognitive dysfunction? *Am J Surg.* 2010;199(6):782–788.

62. Kline RP, Pirraglia E, Cheng H, et al. Surgery and brain atrophy in cognitively normal elderly subjects and subjects diagnosed with mild cognitive impairment. *Anesthesiology.* 2012;116(3):603–612.

63. Hlatky MA, Bacon C, Boothroyd D, et al. Cognitive function 5 years after randomization to coronary angioplasty or coronary artery bypass graft surgery. *Circulation.* 1997;96(9 Suppl):II–11–4; discussion II-5.

64. Cormack F, Shipolini A, Awad WI, et al. A meta-analysis of cognitive outcome following coronary artery bypass graft surgery. *Neurosci Biobehav Rev.* 2012;36(9):2118–2129.

65. Novak V, Hajjar I. The relationship between blood pressure and cognitive function. *Nat Rev Cardiol.* 2010;7(12):686–698.

66. Rudolph JL, Jones RN, Rasmussen LS, Silverstein JH, Inouye SK, Marcantonio ER. Independent vascular and cognitive risk factors for postoperative delirium. *Am J Med.* 2007;120(9):807–813.

67. Selnes OA, Grega MA, Bailey MM, et al. Do management strategies for coronary artery disease influence 6-year cognitive outcomes? *Ann Thorac Surg.* 2009;88(2):445–454.

68. Peters R, Beckett N, Forette F, et al. Incident dementia and blood pressure lowering in the Hypertension in the Very Elderly Trial cognitive function assessment (HYVET-COG): a double-blind, placebo controlled trial. *Lancet Neurol.* 2008;7(8):683–689.

69. Bryson GL, Wyand A. Evidence-based clinical update: general anesthesia and the risk of delirium and postoperative cognitive dysfunction. *Can J Anaesth.* 2006;53(7):669–677.

70. Rasmussen LS, Johnson T, Kuipers HM, et al. Does anaesthesia cause postoperative cognitive dysfunction? A randomised study of regional versus general anaesthesia in 438 elderly patients. *Acta Anaesthesiol Scand.* 2003;47(3):260–266.

71. Sanders RD, Bottle A, Jameson SS, et al. Independent preoperative predictors of outcomes in orthopedic and vascular surgery: the influence of time interval between an acute coronary syndrome or stroke and the operation. *Ann Surg.* 2012;255:901–907.

72. Siepe M, Pfeiffer T, Gieringer A, et al. Increased systemic perfusion pressure during cardiopulmonary bypass is associated with less early postoperative cognitive dysfunction and delirium. *Eur J Cardiothorac Surg.* 2011;40(1):200–207.

73. Whitlock EL, Vannucci A, Avidan MS. Postoperative delirium. *Minerva Anestesiol.* 2011;77(4):448–456.

74. Bryson GL, Wyand A, Wozny D, Rees L, Taljaard M, Nathan H. A prospective cohort study evaluating associations among delirium, postoperative cognitive dysfunction, and apolipoprotein E genotype following open aortic repair. *Can J Anaesth.* 2011;58(3):246–255.

75. Hudetz JA, Patterson KM, Byrne AJ, Pagel PS, Warltier DC. Postoperative delirium is associated with postoperative cognitive dysfunction at one week after cardiac surgery with cardiopulmonary bypass. *Psychol Rep.* 2009;105(3 Pt 1):921–932.

76. Rudolph JL, Marcantonio ER, Culley DJ, et al. Delirium is associated with early postoperative cognitive dysfunction. *Anaesthesia.* 2008;63(9):941–947.

77. Jankowski CJ, Trenerry MR, Cook DJ, et al. Cognitive and functional predictors and sequelae of postoperative delirium in elderly patients undergoing elective joint arthroplasty. *Anesth Analg.* 2011;112(5):1186–1193.

78. Bickel H, Gradinger R, Kochs E, Forstl H. High risk of cognitive and functional decline after postoperative delirium. A three-year prospective study. *Dement Geriatr Cogn Disord.* 2008;26(1):26–31.

79. Kat MG, Vreeswijk R, de Jonghe JF, et al. Long-term cognitive outcome of delirium in elderly hip surgery patients. A prospective matched controlled study over two and a half years. *Dement Geriatr Cogn Disord.* 2008;26(1):1–8.

80. Abildstrom H, Christiansen M, Siersma VD, Rasmussen LS. Apolipoprotein E genotype and cognitive dysfunction after noncardiac surgery. *Anesthesiology.* 2004;101(4):855–861.

81. Avidan MS, Xiong C, Evers AS. Postoperative cognitive decline: the unsubstantiated phenotype. *Anesthesiology.* 2010;113(5):1246–1248; author reply 8–50.

82. Jonsson T, Atwal JK, Steinberg S, et al. A mutation in APP protects against Alzheimer's disease and age-related cognitive decline. *Nature.* 2012;488(7409):96–99.

83. Cibelli M, Fidalgo AR, Terrando N, et al. Role of interleukin-1beta in postoperative cognitive dysfunction. *Ann Neurol.* 2010;68(3):360–368.

84. Cao XZ, Ma H, Wang JK, et al. Postoperative cognitive deficits and neuroinflammation in the hippocampus triggered by surgical trauma are exacerbated in aged rats. *Prog Neuropsychopharmacol Biol Psychiatry.* 2010;34(8):1426–1432.

85. Terrando N, Eriksson LI, Ryu JK, et al. Resolving postoperative neuroinflammation and cognitive decline. *Ann Neurol.* 2011;70(6):986–995.

86. Hudetz JA, Patterson KM, Amole O, Riley AV, Pagel PS. Postoperative cognitive dysfunction after noncardiac surgery: effects of metabolic syndrome. *J Anesth.* 2011;25(3):337–344.

4.

PERIOPERATIVE STROKE

Laurel E. Moore, Lewis B. Morgenstern, and George A. Mashour

INTRODUCTION

Stroke is a devastating complication following surgery, increasing perioperative mortality 2–10 times.[1,2] Despite an incidence similar to perioperative myocardial infarction (MI),[1,3] information regarding prevention and treatment of perioperative stroke is lacking. Furthermore, the physical and emotional impact of perioperative stroke may outweigh that of perioperative MI. From a public health perspective, perioperative stroke increases hospital length of stay[1,4,5] and frequently necessitates chronic care after discharge.[6]

While there are clear premorbid conditions and specific surgical procedures that increase the risk of perioperative stroke, recommendations and guidelines for preventing these events have not yet been developed. Reasons for this are multifactorial and include the low incidence of perioperative stroke and thus difficulty studying it, the absence of accessible biomarkers for postoperative stroke (as compared to troponins or electrocardiogram indicating MI), and the limited treatment options if postoperative stroke is determined to have occurred.

Despite these limitations, the last decade has seen an expanding interest in the relationship between anesthesia and the brain. Neurologic complications of surgery and anesthesia, including postoperative cognitive dysfunction (POCD) and stroke, are being increasingly considered. This chapter will highlight mechanisms and risk factors for perioperative stroke and will summarize the limited recommendations available to reduce the incidence of these events.

In order to be relevant to a wide range of surgical patients, the chapter will focus on perioperative stroke in noncardiac and noncarotid procedures, making comparisons to the cardiac surgery population when relevant. Acute thrombolysis following postoperative stroke will be briefly discussed, although at present the utility of this therapy remains limited because of potential hemorrhagic complications in the postsurgical patient. Stroke after neurosurgical procedures will not be discussed.

INCIDENCE, PREVALENCE, AND OUTCOMES

The majority of perioperative strokes are ischemic and embolic, with fewer than 1% of events being hemorrhagic.[7] By contrast, among nonoperative strokes, 80% are ischemic with the remaining 20% resulting from hemorrhage. The incidence of perioperative stroke ranges from 0.1% to as high as 10%, depending on the type of surgery involved (Table 4.1). This incidence is lower than that of perioperative MI in noncardiac surgery;[6] however, the absence of convenient biomarkers such as troponins or electrocardiograms may limit our ability to diagnose perioperative stroke. Recent data show that most postoperative MIs are asymptomatic[6] and thus would remain undiagnosed without the availability of chemical or electrocardiographic markers of myocardial ischemia. In comparison, surveillance neuroimaging is not routinely performed and assessment of stroke

Table 4.1 INICIDENCE OF PERIOPERATIVE STROKE (30-DAY) IN REPRESENTATIVE SURGICAL POPULATIONS (AGE ≥18 YEARS)

SURGICAL PROCEDURE	INCIDENCE (%)	REFERENCE
Noncardiac non-neurologic	0.1	Mashour[5]
Total hip arthroplasty	0.2	Bateman[14]
Vascular (noncarotid)	0.4–0.8	Axelrod,[4] Sharifpour[1]
Lobectomy/segmental lung resection	0.6	Bateman[14]
Hemicolectomy	0.7	Bateman[14]
Vascular (carotid)	0.9	Harthun[17]
Coronary artery bypass	2.0–3.1	Merie,[15] Roach[16]
Coronary artery bypass and valve replacement	2.2–7.4	Filsoufi,[11] Bucerius[43]
Thoracic endovascular aortic repair (TEVAR)	<1.0–9.4	Melissano[44]
Double and triple valve replacement	9.7	Bucerius[43]

requires recognition of neurologic deterioration. The complexity of detecting subtle mental-status changes or new focal deficits following surgery and anesthesia further confuses our ability to diagnose new cerebral events.

Not surprisingly, procedures associated with an open heart, aortic arch manipulation, and cardiopulmonary bypass, such as valve replacements and thoracic aneurysms, have the highest incidence of postoperative stroke, ranging from 2% to 10% (Table 4.1). Similarly, procedures directly affecting the cerebral circulation, such as carotid endarterectomy, also have high rates of perioperative stroke. Furthermore, these patient populations have associated comorbidities that place them at increased risk for perioperative stroke independent of surgery. Both procedure and comorbidities need to be considered when assessing the global risk for stroke in surgical patients.

In a large study evaluating perioperative stroke in a low-risk patient population, Mashour et al. used the American College of Surgeons National Surgical Quality Improvement Program (ACS-NSQIP) 2005–2008 dataset and found an overall perioperative stroke rate of 0.1% in over 500,000 patients undergoing a broad range of noncardiac and non-neurologic procedures.[5] Using a matched cohort, these investigators showed an 8-fold increase in mortality in those patients suffering postoperative stroke. Also using the ACS-NSQIP database, this time focusing on noncarotid vascular surgery patients (n = 47,650), Sharifpour et al. showed an overall stroke rate of 0.6% in

this high-risk population.[1] Similar to the low-risk cohort, the high-risk population had an overall 3-fold increase in 30-day all-cause mortality in patients suffering perioperative stroke as well as a significant increase in surgical length of stay from 6 to 13 days. Therefore, while the incidence of stroke in noncardiac, non-neurologic patients is well below 1%, perioperative stroke significantly worsens outcome measures such as mortality and hospital length of stay.

When assessing the mechanisms of perioperative stroke, it is important to note that mortality associated with perioperative stroke is increased at least 2-fold compared to strokes occurring in the nonoperative setting.[2] The higher mortality associated with perioperative stroke may in part be due to the unique physiological changes that occur after surgery, including the possibility of existing plaque instability or rupture, activation of the coagulation cascade, decreased fibrinolysis, platelet activation, and endothelial dysfunction[2] (Figure 4.1). Add to these physiological changes the possibility of perioperative hypotension, anemia, and dehydration and it is clear that the etiology of perioperative stroke is multifactorial. Finally, the additional burden of preoperative antiplatelet and anticoagulant therapy discontinuation in this setting may further increase the risk of stroke (Figure 4.2).

Mechanisms of stroke in the cardiac surgery population differ from those in the general surgical population, given the risks associated with cardiopulmonary bypass and manipulation of the heart and thoracic aorta. Patients undergoing cardiac surgery have a markedly increased incidence of watershed infarcts.[8] Gottesman et al. found a 48% incidence of bilateral watershed infarcts in cardiac surgery patients with clinical evidence of stroke.[8] Likewise, Barber et al. found an almost 50% incidence of cerebral ischemia on diffusion-weighted MRI sequences in patients over the first 5 days after open cardiac procedures (e.g., valve replacements),[9] and POCD was associated with these imaging changes. Thus, an additional mechanism of stroke in the cardiac surgery population may be a combination of embolic infarct in watershed regions suggesting poor embolic clearance in areas of hypoperfusion.[9]

Assessing the timing of perioperative stroke is made difficult by the fact that patients who are at greatest risk, for example, those undergoing cardiac and major vascular surgery, often remain sedated and intubated for 12–24 hours after the procedure. Despite these limitations, the timing of perioperative stroke is believed to extend beyond the 48 hours generally associated with the highest risk of perioperative MI.[1,4,6,10] In Sharifpour's noncarotid vascular surgery population, only 15% of strokes occurred in the first 24 hours postprocedure, while 58% occurred within

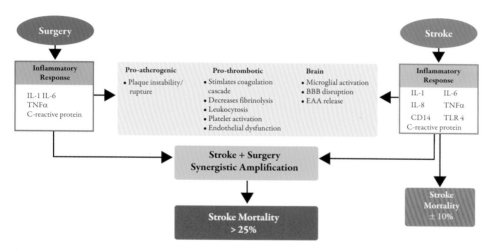

Figure 4.1 The procoagulant and vascular changes associated with surgery and their proposed effects on stroke mortality. BBB, blood–brain barrier; EAA, excitatory amino acid; IL-1, interleukin-1; TNF-α, tumor necrosis factor alpha From Ng et al.,[2] with permission (in progress).

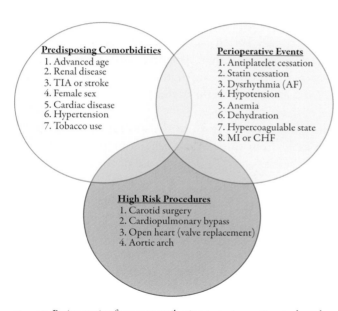

Figure 4.2 Perioperative factors contributing to perioperative stroke risk. Comorbidities and surgical procedures listed are well-established, perioperative events are more conjectural. AF, atrial fibrillation; CHF, congestive heart failure; MI, myocardial infarction; TIA, transient ischemic attack.

the first week.[1] Considering a wider patient population that includes cardiac surgery patients, there is a bimodal distribution with approximately half of strokes presenting within the first 48 hours and the remaining half presenting from postoperative day 2 onward.[7,11] Not surprisingly, early stroke is more common in cardiac patients[7,11] for the reasons described above, although conflicting data support that even in cardiac patients the majority of strokes occur after uneventful neurologic recovery from anesthesia.[10] There are multiple reasons for delayed presentation of perioperative

stroke, including postoperative atrial fibrillation, myocardial infarction, anemia, a surgically induced hypercoagulable state, inflammatory processes, and withdrawal of preoperative antiplatelet agents and/or statins (Figure 4.2). While both immediate and delayed postoperative stroke significantly influences 30-day mortality,[12] there is evidence that cardiac surgery patients suffering delayed stroke have an increased mortality over several years compared to both nonstroke patients and patients suffering immediate postoperative stroke. This suggests that the pathophysiological mechanisms differ between immediate and delayed stroke and that delayed stroke may be indicative of medical conditions that negatively influence survival over time.[12]

In conclusion, while the incidence of postoperative stroke in non-neurologic, noncardiac surgery is <1%, limitations in diagnosing stroke in surgical patients may underestimate this figure. Those patients who are diagnosed with perioperative stroke suffer an increased risk of mortality, a longer hospital stay, and the resultant physical and emotional consequences of stroke.

RISK FACTORS

While there are risk stratification models for perioperative MI and stroke in patients undergoing cardiac surgery,[13] there are few such tools to assess perioperative stroke risk in noncardiac patients. There are, however, known premorbid conditions that have consistently been shown to place patients at increased risk for postoperative stroke (Figure 4.2). In a low-risk surgical population, independent predictors of perioperative stroke include age, recent MI, acute renal failure, history of stroke, dialysis, hypertension, history of transient ischemic attack (TIA), chronic obstructive pulmonary disease, and active tobacco use.[5] Interestingly, body mass index between 35 and 40 was found to be protective in this low-risk population.[5] Atrial fibrillation is not a preoperative condition captured by the ACS-NSQIP data paradigm and thus was not available for analysis in the Mashour study. However, in a large study, Bateman et al. used the Nationwide Inpatient Sample 2000–2004 dataset and identified many of the above factors as well as a history of atrial fibrillation, female sex, and a history of heart failure as risk factors for perioperative stroke.[14] In at least two large studies evaluating perioperative stroke in high-risk noncarotid vascular patients,[1,4] known risk factors such as hypertension, tobacco use, and diabetes have not been found to be independent predictors for stroke, probably because of the high incidence of these comorbidities in this high-risk surgical population.

A prior history of stroke or TIA has been identified as a consistent risk factor for perioperative stroke in multiple studies. Surgical populations in which this is true include cardiac,[13,15] vascular[1,4] and noncardiac non-neurologic procedures.[5,14] Among cardiac surgery patients, as many as 40% of patients suffering postoperative stroke have evidence of chronic cerebral infarction on CT or MRI,[11] while only 10% of these patients reported a history of prior stroke or TIA on preoperative interview, which suggests that history of stroke is a risk factor for which it is difficult to screen. Mechanistically, a history of stroke may indicate pre-existing cerebrovascular disease. Furthermore, prior stroke may leave a region of brain with limited autoregulatory capacity at risk for further injury perioperatively.[15] Not surprisingly, a preoperative history of cerebrovascular disease is a significant predictor of other major adverse cardiac outcomes, such as perioperative MI, congestive heart failure, and death.[3]

Advanced age is another factor that has consistently been shown to place patients at increased risk for perioperative stroke. Furthermore, there is evidence that the proportion of strokes with fatal outcomes also increases with age.[15] Roach et al. published a large prospective study in 1996 documenting an exponential increase in the incidence of major neurologic complications (stroke and coma) as well as more subtle neurologic deficits such as deterioration of intellectual function above the ages of 60–69 years in patients undergoing coronary artery bypass surgery.[16] Since then, age has been supported as a leading risk factor for perioperative stroke in a wide range of surgical procedures, including cardiac,[3,13] vascular,[1,4,17] noncardiac, and nonvascular procedures.[5,14] The elderly present with more advanced atherosclerotic disease, have a higher rate of atrial

fibrillation,[18] and have reduced cerebrovascular reserve compared to that of younger patients,[7] although the clinical relevance of this last factor has recently been called into question.[19] While the mechanism is undoubtedly multifactorial, advanced age clearly remains a major risk factor for perioperative stroke and associated mortality.

A recent area of interest is the apparent increased risk of perioperative stroke in female patients. While women have a lower stroke risk at all ages compared to men (although an increased life-time risk of stroke given longevity), multiple studies demonstrate that in the perioperative setting women are at increased risk for stroke in several surgical populations.[1,7,13,14] Again, the reasons for this are likely to be multifactorial and may include technical difficulties due to smaller vessel size[20] or more advanced disease at presentation in female vascular patients, a higher rate of cardioembolism in women than in men,[21] a reduced sensitivity to antiplatelet therapy,[20,22] and higher thrombotic potential.[20] There has been at least one large study[5] in noncardiac non-neurologic procedures in which female sex was not an independent predictor of stroke. Clearly this is an area of active research. Sex is not a modifiable risk factor, but if the mechanisms of sex-specific differences in stroke rates can be determined, future care might be tailored to improve outcomes for women.

Chronic atrial fibrillation is common among patients undergoing vascular (7.2% of patients preoperatively)[17] and cardiac surgery (10–15% preoperatively).[18] Regardless of the type of surgery, preoperative atrial fibrillation clearly increases the risk of perioperative stroke[14,17,18] as well as short- and long-term mortality.[18] Not only are patients with pre-existing atrial fibrillation at risk for embolic infarcts (particularly with perioperative cessation of anticoagulant therapy), but they are also sicker with a greater incidence of advanced age, history of MI, cerebrovascular disease, and poor left ventricular function. Despite these associations, atrial fibrillation remains an independent predictor of perioperative stroke and death.[17] Patients with chronic atrial fibrillation on warfarin are candidates for bridging therapy with unfractionated or low-molecular-weight heparin perioperatively (see the American College of Chest Physicians Evidence-Based Clinical Practice Guidelines on perioperative antithrombotic therapy[23]). Patients who may be at particular risk for perioperative stroke include those patients in atrial fibrillation with a recent history (less than 6 months) of stroke or TIA.[23] In the last decade several new categories of oral anticoagulant medications have been developed and are being increasingly used in place of vitamin K antagonists for stroke prevention in patients with atrial fibrillation. Two examples include the direct thrombin inhibitors

(DTIs; dabigatran etexilate or Pradoxa® is the first to be FDA approved) and Xa inhibitors (rivaroxaban or Xarelto®, apixaban, betrixaban). Although they have different mechanisms of action, both categories of drugs share the benefits of 1) short half-lives and 2) no requirement for INR surveillance. The Xa inhibitors are particularly short-acting, which may eliminate the need for heparin bridging in high-risk surgical patients. A significant drawback for both drugs is that they have no specific antagonist for rapid reversal. See Douketis (2010) for an excellent review of these new anticoagulants and their perioperative use.[24]

The American Heart Association (AHA) recommendations for continuation of antiplatelet agents perioperatively in patients who have undergone percutaneous coronary intervention (PCI)[25] and the resultant changes in clinical practice are forcing a new look at the continued use of antiplatelet agents in patients with a history of stroke or TIA in the perioperative setting. However, unlike perioperative management of PCI patients on aspirin (ASA), there are limited studies on the perioperative management of patients on ASA for secondary stroke prevention. There are no large studies demonstrating that discontinuation of antiplatelet therapy results in an increase in perioperative strokes, although several case reports suggest this may be the case.[26,27] Acute cerebral events following perioperative ASA cessation occur on average 2 weeks postcessation, though with a wide standard deviation.[26] Much greater surgical attention has been paid to the risk of surgical bleeding in patients who continue antiplatelet therapy perioperatively. Burger et al. did a large review and meta-analysis of studies evaluating the risk of perioperative bleeding in patients who continue to receive low-dose ASA and concluded that perioperative ASA increased the risk of bleeding complications by a factor of 1.5.[26] However, only in transurethral resection of prostate and intracranial procedures were these complications life threatening. Recently, a small retrospective study of patients undergoing transurethral resection of the prostate evaluated the rate of cardiovascular and cerebrovascular complications with perioperative antiplatelet and anticoagulant therapy withdrawal.[27] The majority of patients had been on ASA alone for secondary prevention of MI and stroke. Remarkably, there was a 10% 30-day risk of cardiovascular and cerebrovascular complications (5% 30-day risk of TIA or stroke). An accompanying editorial[28] concluded that in patients receiving antiplatelet or anticoagulant therapy for secondary prevention of cardiac and cerebrovascular complications, a procedure other than transurethral resection of the prostate should be considered so antiplatelet therapy can be continued perioperatively. In summary, there are currently no guidelines for the continuation of antiplatelet

therapy perioperatively, although there are data to support that the abrupt cessation of ASA may place patients at risk for perioperative stroke or TIA. Further work is needed in this area, especially on the additional question of how to manage patients on clopidogrel as a single agent or in combination with ASA.

Unlike antiplatelet therapy, there are good data to support the continuation of statin therapy perioperatively. HMG-CoA reductase inhibitors, or statins, effectively decrease cholesterol, but additional beneficial effects include improved endothelial function, decreased platelet aggregation, and reduced vascular inflammation.[29] It is therefore not surprising that their abrupt removal is associated with a marked increase in the risk of cardiovascular complications, known as "statin withdrawal syndrome."[30] The effect of statin withdrawal is not limited to a loss of beneficial vascular effects but may cause a rebound deterioration of vascular function, including a reduction in endothelial nitric oxide synthase activity, increases in proatherogenic substances, and an increase in platelet aggregation.[30] Vascular surgery patients, particularly those undergoing carotid endarterectomy, are increasingly being administered statins preoperatively as a prophylactic measure for stroke prevention;[31] a 2009 review article in the *Journal of Vascular Surgery* concluded that "prospective randomized trials…cannot be performed anymore…because all vascular patients should receive statin treatment as secondary prevention of cardiovascular disease."[32] While it is premature to suggest that all surgical patients at increased risk for stroke be placed on statins preoperatively, it is also clear that statins should not be discontinued before surgery, and every effort should be made to continue statins on schedule throughout the perioperative period.

β-Blockers have been a mainstay of perioperative MI prevention since the 1990s. However, recent data challenging these assumptions in the noncardiac population and suggesting a possible link between perioperative β-blockers and stroke have resulted in a focused review of the use of perioperative β-blockers by the American College of Cardiology (ACC) and AHA in 2009,[33] and a significant narrowing of the ACC/AHH recommendations for perioperative β-blocker administration. The POISE study, published in 2008,[6] was a prospective double-blinded study designed to investigate the cardioprotective effects of prophylactically administered metoprolol in over 8,000 high-risk patients undergoing noncardiac surgery. Study patients received metoprolol 100 mg orally 2–4 hours before their scheduled procedure, repeated doses according to hemodynamic guidelines for the first 24 hours, and 200 mg orally per day for 30 days postprocedure. While metoprolol effectively reduced the risk of postoperative MI, there was an increase in total mortality (HR 1.33, $p = 0.032$) and stroke (HR 2.17, $p = 0.005$) in patients receiving metoprolol compared to placebo. Not surprisingly, patients receiving metoprolol had a greater incidence of clinically significant intraoperative and postoperative bradycardia and hypotension, which were independent predictors for death (both) and stroke (hypotension only). A large 2008 meta-analysis of 33 randomized controlled trials comparing perioperative β-blocker to placebo (12,306 patients, of whom 8351 were from the POISE study) performed by Bangalore et al.[34] concluded that β-blockers were not associated with any reduction in all-cause mortality, cardiovascular mortality, or heart failure but did cause a reduction in the incidence of nonfatal MI "at the expense of" an increase in the incidence of nonfatal stroke (OR 2.01). It is important to note that with the exclusion of POISE study patients in this meta-analysis, there was no association between β-blockers and perioperative stroke. As with the POISE study, β-blockers were associated with a higher risk of perioperative bradycardia and hypotension in this meta-analysis. Subsequent studies, many by Poldermans' group, have questioned the association between β-blockers and perioperative stroke. Specifically, in two large studies they have no shown no association between chronic β-blocker usage[35] or prophylactic β-blocker administration[36] (started in low doses at least 30 days in advance of surgery and up-titrated to effect) and perioperative stroke. There may be several reasons for these contradictory data. First, metoprolol dosing in the POISE trial was aggressive, resulting in significant hypotension and bradycardia. Furthermore, the acute administration of β-blockers (2–4 hours prior to surgery) does not provide for the nonhemodynamic beneficial effects of β-blockers, such as their anti-inflammatory and plaque stabilization effects, that develop over time.[37] Finally, there may be differential outcomes between β-blocker agents. For example, the high β_1 selectivity of bisoprolol may result in greater cardioprotection than that with less selective agents such as metoprolol.[36] Whether there are differences in stroke potential between β-blockers is unknown. In sum, there is still no clear answer as to whether perioperative β-blockers increase the risk of perioperative stroke. Very recent evidence actually supports that β-blockers may be protective against perioperative stroke (in combination with statins)[38] in coronary artery bypass surgery patients. Clearly the acute discontinuation of β-blockers perioperatively is associated with cardiovascular complications and is to be avoided. The revised 2009 ACC/AHA guidelines conclude that 1) perioperative β-blockers should be continued in patients receiving β-blockers for angina, symptomatic arrhythmias, or hypertension (paraphrased, Class I recommendation), and 2) β-blockers "titrated to heart rate and blood pressure are probably indicated for patients undergoing vascular surgery who are at high cardiac risk owing to coronary artery disease or the finding of cardiac ischemia on preoperative testing" (Class II recommendation).[33]

PREVENTIVE STRATEGIES AND TREATMENT

There are very few data to guide clinicians in the prevention of perioperative stroke. To begin with, most risk factors for perioperative stroke are nonmodifiable (age, sex, renal disease, history of prior stroke, atrial fibrillation, and poor systolic function), although other known risk factors such as tobacco use or hypertension can be optimized preoperatively. The routine use of preoperative carotid duplex scanning to assess for significant stenosis is expensive and not supported by the literature, although there are data to support its use in high-risk patients undergoing cardiac procedures.[39] In terms of procedural factors, certain operations place patients at increased risk for stroke, including procedures involving cardiopulmonary bypass and manipulation of the aortic arch or carotid arteries, and little can be done to alter the technical aspects of these procedures. Recent data in abdominal aortic aneurysm surgery suggest that an endovascular approach might be preferable to an open approach in terms of stroke risk reduction.[1] For most procedures, however, surgical approaches that reduce the risk of perioperative stroke are not clearly defined or are unavailable as an alternative.

The question of whether perioperative blood pressure management can affect the risk of perioperative stroke is critical and remains unanswered. That the majority of perioperative strokes are embolic in nature[7] and that in the noncardiac setting strokes occur greater than 24 hours following surgery[1,7] suggest that intraoperative events are not critical to the incidence of perioperative stroke. Other studies, however, support the opposite conclusion. The POISE study, for example, suggests that perioperative hypotension, including the intraoperative period, did affect the incidence of stroke and death in their large high-risk population.[6] Sabate et al. found a strong association between intraoperative hypotension (defined as ≥20% or ≥20 mmHg decrease in mean arterial pressure for greater than 1 hour) and postoperative major adverse cardiac and cerebrovascular events in a noncardiac population.[3] Bijker et al. found an association between the duration of intraoperative hypotension (defined as ≥30%

reduction in mean arterial pressure) and postoperative stroke in a noncardiac and non-neurosurgical population.[40] The authors suggest that the magnitude of the relationship between intraoperative hypotension and postoperative stroke seen in their study was smaller than that seen in the POISE study. They posit that patients may be at greatest risk for stroke in the immediate postoperative period (during which hemodynamics are not monitored with the same temporal resolution or vigilance as in the operating room) and that intraoperative hypotension may predict postoperative hemodynamic instability and thus postoperative stroke risk.[40] Similarly, there are good data in the cardiac surgery population to support the claim that intraoperative hypotension is associated with worsened neurologic outcomes postoperatively.[8,41] In conclusion, there may be a subset of patients in whom meticulous intraoperative and postoperative blood pressure management is essential, including those patients with a history of TIA or stroke in whom cerebral autoregulation may be abnormal, and patients with poorly controlled hypertension in whom the autoregulatory curve may be right-shifted, placing them at risk for reduced cerebral blood flow at otherwise "normal" mean arterial pressures. For patients deemed to be at risk for perioperative stroke, it seems prudent to maintain intraoperative mean arterial pressure within 20% of preoperative values whenever possible. It is questionable whether the association between intraoperative hypotension and perioperative stroke can ever be studied prospectively, thus the issue may never be fully concluded.

In terms of other preventive strategies to avoid perioperative stroke, there are few recommendations. Statins should be continued in the perioperative period whenever possible, with consideration given to switching to a longer-acting agent such as extended-release fluvastatin when patients will be NPO for a period of time postoperatively. Similarly, patients presenting for surgery on β-blockers should continue to receive them, if only because of the significant cardiovascular risks associated with discontinuation. Further research is mandatory in this area. Finally, and probably least well-supported by clinical studies, patients on ASA for secondary prevention of cardiac and cerebrovascular events should continue ASA perioperatively if the surgical procedure allows. Consideration should be given to a dose of ASA 325 mg by mouth preoperatively for patients who have stopped their antiplatelet therapy preoperatively and are felt to be at high risk for perioperative stroke, again provided the surgery is not associated with high blood loss or catastrophic sequelae to postoperative hematoma formation (e.g., intracranial or spinal surgery).

While there is extensive literature on the management of patients with nonoperative acute ischemic stroke, guidelines for the management of patients with perioperative stroke are essentially nonexistent. The goal of rapid recognition and treatment of perioperative stroke is to minimize brain injury and optimize patient recovery—or, as frequently summarized, "time is brain." The initial challenge in postoperative patients is simply recognizing that the patient has suffered a neurologic insult. This is easily missed in the setting of residual anesthetic effects, pain, sedative administration, and frequent POCD from a multitude of causes, only one of which is cerebral ischemia. In patients felt to be at risk for postoperative stroke, frequently documented neurologic checks are crucial to establishing the timeline for stroke that will dictate time-limited therapies. Table 4.2 displays the Cincinnati Pre-hospital Stroke Scale,[42] an excellent screen for non-neurologists. In *nonoperative* patients, if any one of the three major signs is abnormal, the probability of stroke is 72%; the scale's predictive value in postoperative patients has not been determined, but it serves to demonstrate that a simple neurologic screen might assist in the recognition of perioperative stroke. If stroke is suspected, options for acute intervention in the postoperative setting are limited, given the risk of thrombolytic therapy in the postsurgical patient, although "major surgery or serious trauma within previous 14 days" is only a relative exclusion criterion for intravenous recombinant tissue plasminogen activator (rtPA).[42]

Most hospitals now have a stroke service that specializes in the rapid diagnosis and management of acute ischemic stroke. If a new stroke is suspected, the stroke team should be immediately notified and an emergent head CT obtained to rule out hemorrhage or a well-developed stroke. It is critical that the last known "normal" time be identified, as this will determine what intervention, if any, the patient may receive. MRI should be considered if the

---

Table 4.2 **THE CINCINNATI PRE-HOSPITAL STROKE SCALE**

Facial droop (have patient grimace or show teeth)
• Normal—no droop
• Abnormal—one side of face doesn't move as well as other

Arm drift (patient closes eyes and holds both arms straight out palms up for 10 seconds)
• Normal—both arms move the same
• Abnormal—one arm does not move or drifts down compared to other

Abnormal speech (have the patient say "you can't teach an old dog new tricks")
• Normal—patient uses correct words with no slurring
• Abnormal—patients slurs words, uses the wrong words, or is unable to speak

INTERPRETATION: If any one of these three signs is abnormal, the probability of stroke is 72% *in the nonoperative patient population.* Adapted from *Circulation* 2010:122(Suppl):S818–S828.

timing of the onset of stroke is unclear. If acute ischemic stroke is suspected (and hemorrhage ruled out by CT), permissive hypertension should be considered, although a systolic blood pressure of >185 mmHg or a diastolic blood pressure of >110 mmHg are exclusion criteria for systemic rtPA[42] and might be considered the upper limits for what is acceptable; again, there are no guidelines for the perioperative patient. If an early and significant focal deficit is suspected, strong consideration should be given to emergent cerebral angiography and possible endovascular intervention. Although recent surgery is a relative contraindication to systemic thrombolytic therapy,[42] intra-arterial thrombolysis or mechanical disruption of clot without the use of thrombolytics could be considered in the setting of a potentially devastating stroke, but only if achieved within a limited window of time (3–6 hours depending on stroke severity, interventional technique, and anatomic location of clot). Close hemodynamic monitoring and correction of possible contributory factors such as anemia, hypotension, or hypoxia should be managed aggressively. A complete discussion of the management of acute ischemic stroke is beyond the scope of this chapter; the reader is referred to the 2010 AHA Guidelines for Cardiopulmonary Resuscitation and Emergency Cardiovascular Care Part II: Adult Stroke[42] for a more thorough discussion of current guidelines and management options.

Patients who have suffered a perioperative stroke die from a number of etiologies related to extended hospitalization and immobilization, including respiratory insufficiency, aspiration, MI, thromboembolism, pneumonia, and sepsis. Excellent nursing care, supportive medical care including tight glucose control and hemodynamic monitoring, and referral to physical medicine and rehabilitation experts should be standard care for these patients.

CURRENT GUIDELINES AND RECOMMENDATIONS

There are currently no formal guidelines for the management of perioperative stroke.

CONCLUSION

Perioperative stroke is an uncommon but potentially devastating complication of surgery. Because most premorbid conditions that predispose to perioperative stroke are nonmodifiable, further research is needed to evaluate intraoperative and postoperative factors that are potentially modifiable

in order to reduce the incidence of stroke in surgical patients. Most medical institutions now have "stroke teams" that rapidly respond to in-house strokes and help determine candidacy for acute stroke interventions. Emergent consultation with the stroke service at the first sign of a new neurologic deficit is crucial. Finally, we need to develop and implement guidelines for the perioperative management of patients with a history of stroke or TIA as well as those who suffer the potentially devastating complication of postoperative stroke.

CONFLICT OF INTEREST STATEMENT

L.E.M., L.B.M., and G.A.M. have no conflicts of interest to disclose.

REFERENCES

1. Sharifpour M, Moore LE, Shanks A, et al. Incidence, predictors, and outcomes of perioperative stroke in noncarotid major vascular surgery. *Anesth Analg.* 2012; October 31. [Epub ahead of print]
2. Ng JL, Chan MT, Gelb AW. Perioperative stroke in noncardiac, nonneurosurgical surgery. *Anesthesiology.* 2011;115:879–890.
3. Sabate S, Mases A, Guilera N, et al. Incidence and predictors of major perioperative adverse cardiac and cerebrovascular events in non-cardiac surgery. *Br J Anaesth.* 2011;107:879–890.
4. Axelrod DA, Stanley JC, Upchurch GR, Jr., et al. Risk for stroke after elective noncarotid vascular surgery. *J Vasc Surg.* 2004;39:67–72.
5. Mashour GA, Shanks AM, Kheterpal S. Perioperative stroke and associated mortality after noncardiac, nonneurologic surgery. *Anesthesiology.* 2011;114:1289–1296.
6. Devereaux PJ, Yang H, Yusuf S, et al. Effects of extended-release metoprolol succinate in patients undergoing non-cardiac surgery (POISE trial): a randomised controlled trial. *Lancet.* 2008;371:1839–1847.
7. Selim M. Perioperative stroke. *N Engl J Med.* 2007;356:706–713.
8. Gottesman RF, Sherman PM, Grega MA, et al. Watershed strokes after cardiac surgery: diagnosis, etiology, and outcome. *Stroke.* 2006;37:2306–2311.
9. Barber PA, Hach S, Tippett LJ, Ross L, Merry AF, Milsom P. Cerebral ischemic lesions on diffusion-weighted imaging are associated with neurocognitive decline after cardiac surgery. *Stroke.* 2008;39:1427–1433.
10. Hogue CW, Jr., Murphy SF, Schechtman KB, Davila-Roman VG. Risk factors for early or delayed stroke after cardiac surgery. *Circulation.* 1999;100:642–647.
11. Filsoufi F, Rahmanian PB, Castillo JG, Bronster D, Adams DH. Incidence, topography, predictors and long-term survival after stroke in patients undergoing coronary artery bypass grafting. *Ann Thorac Surg.* 2008;85:862–870.
12. Hedberg M, Boivie P, Engstrom KG. Early and delayed stroke after coronary surgery—an analysis of risk factors and the impact on short- and long-term survival. *Eur J Cardiothorac Surg.* 2011;40:379–387.
13. Charlesworth DC, Likosky DS, Marrin CA, et al. Development and validation of a prediction model for strokes after coronary artery bypass grafting. *Ann Thorac Surg.* 2003;76:436–443.
14. Bateman BT, Schumacher HC, Wang S, Shaefi S, Berman MF. Perioperative acute ischemic stroke in noncardiac and nonvascular surgery: incidence, risk factors, and outcomes. *Anesthesiology.* 2009;110:231–238.

15. Merie C, Kober L, Olsen PS, Andersson C, Jensen JS, Torp-Pedersen C. Risk of stroke after coronary artery bypass grafting: effect of age and comorbidities. *Stroke.* 2012;43:38–43.
16. Roach GW, Kanchuger M, Mangano CM, et al. Adverse cerebral outcomes after coronary bypass surgery. Multicenter study of Perioperative Ischemia Research Group and the Ischemia Research and Education Foundation Investigators. *N Engl J Med.* 1996;335:1857–1863.
17. Harthun NL, Stukenborg GJ. Atrial fibrillation is associated with increased risk of perioperative stroke and death from carotid endarterectomy. *J Vasc Surg.* 2010;51:330–336.
18. Attaran S, Shaw M, Bond L, Pullan MD, Fabri BM. A comparison of outcome in patients with preoperative atrial fibrillation and patients in sinus rhythm. *Ann Thorac Surg.* 2011;92:1391–1395.
19. Burkhart CS, Rossi A, Dell-Kuster S, et al. Effect of age on intraoperative cerebrovascular autoregulation and near-infrared spectroscopy-derived cerebral oxygenation. *Br J Anaesth.* 2011;107:742–748.
20. den Hartog AG, Algra A, Moll FL, de Borst GJ. Mechanisms of gender-related outcome differences after carotid endarterectomy. *J Vasc Surg.* 2010;52:1062–1071, e1–e6.
21. Forster A, Gass A, Kern R, et al. Gender differences in acute ischemic stroke: etiology, stroke patterns and response to thrombolysis. *Stroke.* 2009;40:2428–2432.
22. Cavallari LH, Helgason CM, Brace LD, Viana MA, Nutescu EA. Sex difference in the antiplatelet effect of aspirin in patients with stroke. *Ann Pharmacother.* 2006;40:812–817.
23. Douketis JD, Berger PB, Dunn AS, et al. The perioperative management of antithrombotic therapy: American College of Chest Physicians Evidence-Based Clinical Practice Guidelines (8th edition). *Chest.* 2008;133:299S–339S.
24. Douketis JD. Pharmacologic properties of the new oral anticoagulants: a clinician-oriented review with a focus on perioperative management. *Curr Pharm Des.* 2010;16:3436–3441.
25. Fleisher LA, Beckman JA, Brown KA, et al. 2009 ACCF/AHA focused update on perioperative beta-blockade incorporated into the ACC/AHA 2007 guidelines on perioperative cardiovascular evaluation and care for noncardiac surgery. *J Am Coll Cardiol.* 2009;54:e13–e118.
26. Burger W, Chemnitius JM, Kneissl GD, Rucker G. Low-dose aspirin for secondary cardiovascular prevention—cardiovascular risks after its perioperative withdrawal versus bleeding risks with its continuation—review and meta-analysis. *J Intern Med.* 2005;257:399–414.
27. Taylor K, Filgate R, Guo DY, Macneil F. A retrospective study to assess the morbidity associated with transurethral prostatectomy in patients on antiplatelet or anticoagulant drugs. *BJU Int.* 2011;108(Suppl 2):45–50.
28. Woo HH. We should cease offering turp in favour of alternative surgery options for anticoagulated patients. *BJU Int.* 2011;108(Suppl 2):50.
29. Paciaroni M, Bogousslavsky J. Statins and stroke prevention. *Expert Rev Cardiovasc Ther.* 2009;7:1231–1243.
30. Pineda A, Cubeddu LX. Statin rebound or withdrawal syndrome: does it exist? *Curr Atheroscler Rep.* 2011;13:23–30.
31. Perler BA. Should statins be given routinely before carotid endarterectomy? *Perspect Vasc Surg Endovasc Ther.* 2007;19:240–245.
32. Stalenhoef AF. The benefit of statins in non-cardiac vascular surgery patients. *J Vasc Surg.* 2009;49:260–265.
33. Fleischmann KE, Beckman JA, Buller CE, et al. 2009 ACCF/AHA focused update on perioperative beta-blockade. *J Am Coll Cardiol.* 2009;54:2102–2128.
34. Bangalore S, Wetterslev J, Pranesh S, Sawhney S, Gluud C, Messerli FH. Perioperative beta blockers in patients having non-cardiac surgery: a meta-analysis. *Lancet.* 2008;372:1962–1976.
35. van Lier F, Schouten O, van Domburg RT, et al. Effect of chronic beta-blocker use on stroke after noncardiac surgery. *Am J Cardiol.* 2009;104:429–433.
36. van Lier F, Schouten O, Hoeks SE, et al. Impact of prophylactic beta-blocker therapy to prevent stroke after noncardiac surgery. *Am J Cardiol.* 2010;105:43–47.
37. Poldermans D, Schouten O, van Lier F, et al. Perioperative strokes and beta-blockade. *Anesthesiology.* 2009;111:940–945.
38. Bouchard D, Carrier M, Demers P, et al. Statin in combination with beta-blocker therapy reduces postoperative stroke after coronary artery bypass graft surgery. *Ann Thorac Surg.* 2011;91:654–659.
39. Cornily JC, Le Saux D, Vinsonneau U, et al. Assessment of carotid artery stenosis before coronary artery bypass surgery. Is it always necessary? *Arch Cardiovasc Dis.* 2011;104:77–83.
40. Bijker JB, Persoon S, Peelen LM, et al. Intraoperative hypotension and perioperative ischemic stroke after general surgery: a nested case-control study. *Anesthesiology.* 2012;116:658–664.
41. Gottesman RF, Hillis AE, Grega MA, et al. Early postoperative cognitive dysfunction and blood pressure during coronary artery bypass graft operation. *Arch Neurol.* 2007;64:1111–1114.
42. Jauch EC, Cucchiara B, Adeoye O, et al. Part 11: adult stroke: 2010 American Heart Association Guidelines for Cardiopulmonary Resuscitation and Emergency Cardiovascular Care. *Circulation.* 2010;122:S818–S828.
43. Bucerius J, Gummert JF, Borger MA et al. Stroke after cardiac surgery: a risk factor analysis of 16,184 consecutive adult patients. *Ann Thorac Surg.* 2003;75:472–478
44. Melissano G, Tshomba Y, Bertoglio L, Rinaldi E, Chiesa R. Analysis of stroke after TEVAR involving the aortic arch. *Eur J Vasc Endovasc Surg.* 2012;Mar;43(3):269–275.

5.

SEIZURES

Adam D. Niesen, Adam K. Jacob, and Sandra L. Kopp

INTRODUCTION TO THE CLINICAL PROBLEM

Postoperative seizures are rare events that may be challenging to evaluate, diagnose, or manage. It is important to recognize and respond to neurologic changes occurring in the perioperative period. Specifically, perioperative physicians should have a clear comprehension of the pathophysiology of and risk factors for seizures as well as the common treatments. Neurosurgical patients represent a unique subset of perioperative patients with distinctive characteristics and challenges that usually do not apply to the general perioperative population in regard to perioperative seizures. Therefore, this chapter will not discuss seizure activity in neurosurgical patients.

By definition, a seizure is the clinical manifestation of abnormally hyperexcitable cortical neurons. Although seizures are commonly thought of in the context of epilepsy syndromes, isolated seizure activity may result from a variety of acute conditions throughout a person's lifetime (e.g., fever, trauma, electrolyte disturbances, infection, alcohol withdrawal). In the general population, there is an 8–10% lifetime risk of experiencing a single seizure and a 3% risk of developing a persistent seizure disorder.[1,2] Therefore, a significant proportion of patients with previous seizure activity will present for anesthesia and surgery at some time in their lives.

Seizure types are classified into two broad categories based on clinical and electroencephalography (EEG) data: partial and generalized (Table 5.1). Partial, or focal, seizures originate and remain in a limited area of the brain and are subclassifed on the basis of consciousness during seizure activity. Consciousness is impaired during complex partial seizures, while consciousness is preserved during simple partial seizures. Further subclassification is based on the clinical signs and symptoms of the partial seizure. Generalized seizures involve both cerebral hemispheres and typically do not present with focal features. Consciousness is always impaired and the seizure may manifest with motor symptoms (convulsive) or without motor symptoms (nonconvulsive).

In general, many factors may contribute to a change in seizure threshold, including antiepileptic medication noncompliance, altered timing of antiepileptic medication administration, altered gastrointentinal absorption of these medications, electrolyte distrubances, anesthetic agents, metabolic derangements, drug and alcohol withdrawl, and sleep deprivation.[3–6] These conditions regularly occur during the perioperative period or while patients are hospitalized. Excluding neurosurgical procedures, a specific type of surgical procedure has not been associated with perioperative seizures.[7] However, seizures following cardiac surgery are well-known, serious complications, and the incidence is probably underestimated.[8] It is thought that seizure activity during or after cardiac surgery is likely a marker of both focal and global cerebral ischemic events. In infants and children, early seizures following cardiac surgery are indicative of central nervous system injury and have been linked to adverse neurologic outcomes.[9]

Table 5.1 **SEIZURE CLASSIFICATION**

SEIZURE TYPE	FEATURES
Generalized	
Absence	Brief episodes of staring, unawareness, unresponsiveness. May occur anytime, often with hyperventilation. No warning before seizure, completely alert immediately after seizure.
Atypical absence	Brief episodes of staring, often somewhat responsive. Hard to distinguish from the person's usual behavior. Unlike other absence seizures, cannot be produced by hyperventilation.
Myoclonic	Brief, sudden, involuntary, shock-like muscle contraction arising from the central nervous system that causes either generalized or focal clonic jerks. This type occurs in a variety of epilepsy syndromes with different characteristics.
Atonic	Very brief sudden loss of tone, which may be limited to eye blinks or head drops but can involve the entire body. A myoclonic jerk may precede or accompany the seizure.
Tonic	Episodes of increased muscle tone/stiffening movements in the body, arms, or legs. Consciousness is usually preserved. Seizures often occur during sleep, affecting both sides of the body.
Clonic	Rapidly alternating contraction and relaxation of a muscle. Movements cannot be stopped by restraining or repositioning the arms or legs.
Tonic-clonic	Formerly known as "grand mal" seizure. Often idiopathic. It is usually preceded by an aura, then progresses to the tonic and clonic phases, followed by postictal period with somnolence, confusion, and amnesia.
Partial	
Simple partial	Brief episodes of varying symptoms (motor, sensory, autonomic, psychic), depending on which specific region of the brain is affected. Often the focus is located in the temporal lobe and/or hippocampus. Often there is a subjective experience (auras, sensory hallucinations). Consciousness is retained. This type of seizure is often a precursor to larger seizures.
Complex partial	Usually preceded by an aura (e.g., simple partial seizure), larger portion of the brain is affected, causing loss of consciousness. The person may display automatisms such as lip smacking, chewing, or swallowing. The seizure most commonly originates in the temporal lobe.
Secondary generalized	Begins as a simple partial or complex partial seizure, abnormal electrical activity spreads to both cerebral hemispheres. This type commonly results in generalized seizure with tonic-clonic features.

Nonconvulsive seizures may be frequently missed, although they may contribute to prolonged depression of consciousness and possibly increased morbidity and mortality.

INCIDENCE, PREVALENCE, AND OUTCOMES

As discussed earlier, there is an estimated 8–10% lifetime risk of experiencing a single seizure and a 3% risk of developing a persistent seizure disorder.[1,2] The incidence of epilepsy is higher in the intellectually and developmentally disabled population, and there is increased morbidity and mortality in children with seizures and neurologic deficits.[10,11] These patients tend to have more frequent seizures and often require anesthesia for routine procedures (e.g., radiology exams, dental exams and treatment) or for procedures related to trauma incurred during a seizure.[12]

A multicenter prospective cohort study in Thailand was the first large-scale study to estimate the incidence of perioperative seizures in the general population. They reported an incidence of postoperative seizure of 3.1 per 10,000 for all patients undergoing all surgical (including neurosurgical procedures) and anesthesia types, but the incidence of postoperative seizure in patients with an underlying seizure disorder was not reported.[13]

Two subsequent cohort studies have evaluated the risk of perioperative seizures among patients with a known seizure disorder. The first, a population-based study, examined the incidence of seizures in patients with epilepsy undergoing general anesthesia for procedures other than neurosurgical or invasive neurodiagnostic procedures.[14] Seizures were observed in 2% of patients, with no adverse effects reported after receiving general anesthesia. Five of the six identified seizures occurred in children under 13 years of age. Thus, the incidence in adults was 0.8% and the incidence in children was 3%. A subsequent retrospective cohort study reported an overall frequency of perioperative seizures of 3.4% (95% confidence interval, 2.2%–5.2%) among patients with a known seizure disorder who received any anesthetic.[7] The perioperative period was defined as the time from surgery until dismissal from the hospital or 3 days after the anesthetic, whichever time period was longer. The frequency of preoperative seizures ($p < 0.001$) and the timing of the most recent seizure ($p < 0.001$) were both found to be significantly related to the likelihood of experiencing a perioperative seizure. As the number of antiepileptic medications increased, so did the frequency of perioperative seizures ($p < 0.001$). Neither the type of surgery nor the type of anesthetic (general anesthesia, regional anesthesia, or monitored anesthesia care) affected the frequency of perioperative seizures in this patient population. The authors concluded that most perioperative seizures in patients with a pre-existing seizure disorder are likely related to the patient's underlying condition.

The association of anesthesia type and perioperative seizure risk was further evaluated in a group of patients with a history of a seizure disorder who underwent regional anesthesia.[15] In this retrospective review, 24 patients (5.8%) with history of a seizure disorder undergoing a regional anesthetic experienced seizure activity during the postoperative hospital course. None of the seizures were conclusively linked to the regional technique. Upon examination of the time interval between local anesthetic injection and/or termination of the infusion and the event, it was determined that the regional anesthetic was neither the primary etiology nor a contributing factor for the seizure in 19 of 24 patients. In the remaining five patients, perioperative seizure activity was characteristic of their usual seizure, although local anesthetic toxicity could not be absolutely excluded as a contributing factor. Similarly, the timing of the most recent (preoperative) seizure was found to be significantly related to the likelihood of experiencing a postoperative seizure ($p < 0.001$). Again, the conclusion was similar: patients with more frequent seizures preoperatively were more likely to experience a seizure in the postoperative period.

Postoperative neurologic deficit, including seizure, is a well-known complication after cardiac surgery. The estimated incidence of seizures following cardiac surgery ranges from approximately 0.4% to 3.8%.[8,16–18] A recent review of 2,578 consecutive patients undergoing cardiac surgery at a single institution was performed to help elucidate the predictors and outcomes of seizures in this patient population.[8] Of the 31 (1.2%) patients that experienced a postoperative seizure, 71% were classified as generalized tonic–clonic, 26% simple/complex partial, and 3% status epilepticus. The incidence also varied according to procedure (coronary bypass 0.1%, isolated valve 1%, valve/coronary bypass 3%, aorta 5%; $p < 0.001$). Patients who seized had nearly a 5-fold higher operative mortality than that of patients who did not experience a seizure. It appears that seizures in adult patients undergoing cardiac surgery are predictors of permanent neurologic deficit and increased operative mortality.[8] Heart transplant patients have an even higher incidence of postoperative seizures, at approximately 4.8%.

RISK FACTORS

Common provocative factors for seizure activity in patients with or without a seizure disorder include fever, head injury, excessive alcohol intake, withdrawal from alcohol or drugs, hypoglycemia, electrolyte disturbances, intracranial infection or hemorrhage, ischemic stroke, and drugs that may lower the seizure threshold (e.g., tramadol, theophylline, baclofen, ketamine, meperidine).[19] In addition, there are several factors that may increase the risk for seizure activity in patients with a seizure disorder (Table 5.2), including changes in antiepileptic drug levels, fatigue, stress, sleep deprivation, menstruation, and excessive alcohol intake.[3,4,20] Stress and sleep deprivation are particularly common in hospitalized patients. In addition, many situations arise in the perioperative period that can affect antiepileptic drug levels. These include but are not limited to preoperative medication noncompliance, changes in dosing schedule, interaction with other perioperative medications, anesthetic exposure, and changes in gastrointestinal motility leading to delayed absorption and reduced bioavailability.[4,6] In particular, when patients are advised to take nothing by mouth (NPO) preoperatively, they may omit their scheduled doses of antiepileptic medications. This is exacerbated postoperatively in patients who are not allowed to take oral medications because of their surgical procedure or are unable to tolerate oral intake because of nausea and vomiting. Decreased antiepileptic drug serum levels may contribute to perioperative seizure activity.[5]

In a retrospective review of patients with a seizure disorder undergoing anesthesia, over 40% of patients who experienced a perioperative seizure were felt to have changing drug levels as a contributing factor.[7] The therapeutic level for antiepileptic medications must be interpreted individually, as it is a value that depends on the individual patient and the timing of the blood draw. It is not uncommon for an individual patient's therapeutic level to lie outside of the laboratory standard therapeutic range. Furthermore, antiepileptic drugs are subject to many drug–drug interactions and fluctuations due to substitution of generic antiepileptics for brand-name drugs, or substitution of a generic formulation from one manufacturer for the same generic drug produced by a different manufacturer.[21] Drugs such as phenytoin, phenobarbital, and carbamazepine alter the hepatic metabolism of many drugs and induce cytochrome P450 enzyme activity. In addition, a number of medications routinely used in the perioperative period can affect the seizure threshold or have significant interactions with antiepileptic drugs.[22] Patients requiring multiple medications for seizure control present a particular challenge, as they are at a greater risk of seizure

Table 5.2 RISK FACTORS ASSOCIATED WITH PERIOPERATIVE SEIZURE ACTIVITY

FACTORS ASSOCIATED WITH INCREASED FREQUENCY OF POSTOPERATIVE SEIZURES	FACTORS NOT ASSOCIATED WITH INCREASED FREQUENCY OF POSTOPERATIVE SEIZURES
Patients with pre-existing seizure disorder: • More frequent seizure activity at baseline • Increasing number of antiepileptic medications • Short time between last seizure and surgery • Younger age Patients undergoing cardiac surgery: • Cerebral ischemic event • Preoperative cardiac arrest • Open chamber procedure • Deep hypothermic circulatory arrest • Bypass time >150 minutes • Aortic calcification or atheroma • Critically ill perioperative state • Tranexamic acid use	• Anesthetic technique (general, regional, monitored anesthesia care) • Type of surgery (not including neurologic or cardiac surgery)

recurrence when medications are withdrawn or when their dosage is reduced.[23] Not surprisingly, as the number of baseline antiepileptic medications increases, the risk of perioperative seizure activity also increases.[7,15] Consultation with a neurologist may be necessary to formulate the most effective plan for these patients in the perioperative period. Patients whose last seizure occurred close to the time of admission and those with more frequent seizure activity at baseline are more likely to suffer a seizure in the perioperative period.

Risk factors for seizures following cardiac surgery include focal or global ischemia following hypoperfusion, emboli (particulate or air), metabolic derangements, and drug reactions.[8] In addition, deep hypothermic circulatory arrest, aortic calcification or atheroma, and critical perioperative state have been identified as risk factors.[8] Tranexamic acid usage has been linked to seizures in patients undergoing cardiac surgery.[16–18,24] Tranexamic acid competitively binds to GABAA receptors, resulting in reduced inhibitory activity and increased neuronal excitation.[24] The seizures linked to tranexamic acid appear to occur early in the postoperative period, are typically generalized tonic-clonic, and are relatively easy to treat. Following heart transplantation, posterior reversible encephalopathy syndrome (PRES) caused by therapeutic cyclosporin is an additional cause of seizures in this patient population.[25] Symptoms tend to reverse after changing the immunosuppressant medications.

PREVENTIVE STRATEGIES AND TREATMENT

Logically, the most effective strategy to prevent a perioperative seizure is to avoid, or at least optimize, any and all possible known perioperative risk factors that might lower the patient's seizure threshold. This largely depends on the patient's baseline health status and the procedure that he or she is undergoing. Unless surgery is urgent or emergent, all electrolyte or metabolic derangements should be corrected preoperatively. In patients with a pre-existing seizure disorder who are taking antiepileptic medications, preoperative medication noncompliance or missed doses due to NPO status may result in decreased antiepileptic drug levels. Therefore, the patient's usual antiepileptic medication regimen should be followed as closely as possible the day of surgery, especially for those patients with frequent or recent seizures. Furthermore, it is important to maintain an inpatient dosing regimen as close as possible to the outpatient regimen. This can be particularly challenging, as a number of antiepileptics do not have a parenteral formulation and the interpretation of blood levels may be difficult for practitioners unfamiliar with these medications.

Preventive strategies aimed at optimizing intraoperative cerebral protection play a role in improving outcomes in patients who are at risk.[8] Intraoperative use of drugs known to induce epileptiform EEG activity (e.g., etomidate, sevoflurane) should be avoided unless there is strong indication of their superiority over alternative anesthetic options. Furthermore, consideration should be given to prophylaxis with agents that help suppress neuronal excitatory activity (e.g., benzodiazepines, gabapentin).[26]

The anesthesiologist should also be prepared to treat seizure activity in the perioperative setting, particularly in those patients who have frequent seizures at baseline and those who have experienced seizure activity close to the time of admission. The management of patients experiencing postoperative seizures is focused on administration of oxygen, management of hemodynamics, and seizure termination. In addition to treatment with GABAergic agents such as benzodiazepines, the sodium channel blocker phenytoin and the mixed-action agent valproate are recommended for treatment of perioperative seizures. Valproic acid can be infused rapidly and rarely causes hypotension; it also has very little sedative effect and is long-acting. Newer intravenous anticonvulsant drugs (valproic acid, levetiracetam) have helped to minimize the undesired side effects (hypotension, bradycardia, cardiac arrest) associated with phenytoin and fosphenytoin.

Early head computed tomography (CT) has been indicated to identify treatable pathology. With aggressive management, the outcome is generally good, with little residual neurologic impairment. In status epilepticus, continuous seizure activity occurs for 5 minutes or longer, or two or more seizures are clustered together without full recovery of consciousness between seizures. At this point, neuronal injury may have already occurred and spontaneous termination of the seizure is unlikely.[27]

CURRENT GUIDELINES AND RECOMMENDATIONS

Patients with a new diagnosis of seizures or poorly controlled seizures require evaluation to determine the cause of the seizure. Ideally, this should occur before the patient presents for an anesthetic. The anesthetic management of a patient with a history of seizures is influenced more by the *cause* of the seizure than the fact that the patient has had a seizure. Seizures that occur intraoperatively may be related to the anesthetic technique, whereas seizures that occur postoperatively are generally related to the patient's underlying seizure disorder rather than anesthetic management. Anesthetic agents such as propofol, thiopental, benzodiazepines, and volatile anesthetics (excluding enflurane and sevoflurane) cause a dose-dependent increase in the seizure threshold. Agents such as alfentanil, remifentanil, and methohexital have been shown to reduce the seizure threshold.

There are several different types of antiepileptic drugs used to control patient's seizures. Most anticonvulsants (phenytoin, phenobarbital, and carbamazepine) induce the cytochrome P450 system, which can lead to resistance to neuromuscular blocking agents. Individual patient preoperative laboratory testing will depend on the specific side effects of their antiepileptic agent. A complete blood count and platelet count in addition to an electrolyte panel are the most commonly obtained preoperative tests. Valproic acid has been shown to interfere with platelet count and function in addition to reducing fibrinogen and von Willebrand factor, thus interfering with hemostasis.[28] Preoperative coagulation profiles are recommended for patients taking valproic acid.

Despite the potential interactions, most authorities believe that it is essential to continue patients on their usual antiepileptic medication. This includes encouraging patients to take their usual morning dose with a sip of water in the preoperative period. For patients who are unable to take oral medications perioperatively, there are several parenteral options (e.g., phenytoin, valproate, levetiracetam,

and phenobarbital). In addition, some medications are available as a suspension for nasogastric tube administration. Obviously, these medication adjustments should be directed by a neurologist familiar with the patient's underlying seizure disorder.

CONCLUSION

Seizures are uncommon events in the perioperative period in the general population. However, patients with a pre-existing seizure disorder and cardiac surgical patients are at higher risk of perioperative seizures. Patients who experience more frequent seizures at baseline require multiple medications for daily seizure control, and patients whose most recent seizure occurred close to the date of surgery are at higher risk for postoperative seizure activity. In cardiac surgical patients, cerebral ischemia, long bypass times, deep hypothermic circulatory arrest, aortic calcification or atheroma, critically ill perioperative state, and the use of tranexamic acid are all risk factors for seizure activity. Sleep deprivation, stress, electrolyte disturbances, and alteration of the patient's typical antiepileptic regimen can also contribute to an increased rate of perioperative seizures. However, with close attention to maintenance of the patient's home antiepileptic regimen, early recognition of seizure activity, and prompt treatment, the negative consequences of perioperative seizure activity can be minimized.

CONFLICT OF INTEREST STATEMENT

A.J. and S.K. have no conflicts of interest to disclose.

REFERENCES

1. Hauser WA, Rich SS, Annegers JF, Anderson VE. Seizure recurrence after a 1st unprovoked seizure: An extended follow-up. *Neurology.* 1990;40(8):1163–1170.
2. Hauser WA, Annegers JF, Kurland LT. Incidence of epilepsy and unprovoked seizures in Rochester, Minnesota: 1935-1984. *Epilepsia.* 1993;34(3):453–468.
3. Delanty N, Vaughan CJ, French JA. Medical causes of seizures. *Lancet.* 1998;352(9125):383–390.
4. Paul F, Veauthier C, Fritz G, et al. Perioperative fluctuations of lamotrigine serum levels in patients undergoing epilepsy surgery. *Seizure.* 2007;16(6):479–484.
5. Specht U, Elsner H, May TW, Schimichowski B, Thorbecke R. Postictal serum levels of antiepileptic drugs for detection of noncompliance. *Epilepsy Behav.* 2003;4(5):487–495.
6. Tan JH, Wilder-Smith E, Lim ECH, Ong BKC. Frequency of provocative factors in epileptic patients admitted for seizures: a prospective study in Singapore. *Seizure.* 2005;14(7):464–469.

7. Niesen AD, Jacob AK, Aho LE, et al. Perioperative seizures in patients with a history of a seizure disorder. *Anesth Analg.* 2010;111(3):729–735.

8. Goldstone AB, Bronster DJ, Anyanwu AC, et al. Predictors and outcomes of seizures after cardiac surgery: a multivariable analysis of 2,578 patients. *Ann Thorac Surg.* 2011;91(2):514–518.

9. Bellinger DC, Jonas RA, Rappaport LA, et al. Developmental and neurologic status of children after heart surgery with hypothermic circulatory arrest or low-flow cardiopulmonary bypass. *N Engl J Med.* 1995;332(9):549–555.

10. Brorson LO, Wranne L. Long-term prognosis in childhood epilepsy: survival and seizure prognosis. *Epilepsia.* 1987;28(4):324–330.

11. Forsgren L, Hauser WA, Olafsson E, Sander JWAS, Sillanpää M, Tomson T. Mortality of epilepsy in developed countries: a review. *Epilepsia.* 2005;46(Suppl. 11):18–27.

12. Ren WH. Anesthetic management of epileptic pediatric patients. *Int Anesthesiol Clinics.* 2009;47(3):101–116.

13. Akavipat P, Rungreungvanich M, Lekprasert V, Srisawasdi S. The Thai Anesthesia Incidents Study (THAI Study) of perioperative convulsion. *J Med Assoc Thai.* 2005;88(Suppl. 7):S106–S112.

14. Benish SM, Cascino GD, Warner ME, Worrell GA, Wass CT. Effect of general anesthesia in patients with epilepsy: a population-based study. *Epilepsy Behav.* 2009;17(1):87–89.

15. Kopp SL, Wynd KP, Horlocker TT, Hebl JR, Wilson JL. Regional blockade in patients with a history of a seizure disorder. *Anesth Analg.* 2009;109(1):272–278.

16. Martin K, Wiesner G, Breuer T, Lange R, Tassani P. The risks of aprotinin and tranexamic acid in cardiac surgery: a one-year follow-up of 1188 consecutive patients. *Anesth Analg.* 2008;107(6):1783–1790.

17. Murkin JM, Falter F, Granton J, Young B, Burt C, Chu M. High-dose tranexamic acid is associated with nonischemic clinical seizures in cardiac surgical patients. *Anesth Analg.* 2010;110(2):350–353.

18. Roach GW, Kanchuger M, Mangano CM, et al. Adverse cerebral outcomes after coronary bypass surgery. Multicenter study of Perioperative Ischemia Research Group and the Ischemia Research and Education Foundation Investigators. *N Engl J Med.* 1996;335(25):1857–1863.

19. Pohlmann-Eden B, Beghi E, Camfield C, Camfield P. The first seizure and its management in adults and children. *BMJ.* 2006;332(7537):339–342.

20. Sokic D, Ristic AJ, Vojvodic N, Jankovic S, Sindjelic AR. Frequency, causes and phenomenology of late seizure recurrence in patients with juvenile myoclonic epilepsy after a long period of remission. *Seizure.* 2007;16(6):533–537.

21. Tatum WO. Antiepileptic drugs: adverse effects and drug interactions. *Continuum (Minneapolis Minn).* 2010;16(3):136–158.

22. Cheng MA, Tempelhoff R. Anesthesia and epilepsy. *Curr Opin Anaesthesiol.* 1999;12(5):523–528.

23. Barton G, Hicks E, Patterson VH, et al. Randomised study of antiepileptic drug withdrawal in patients in remission. *Lancet.* 1991;337(8751):1175–1180.

24. Manji RA, Grocott HP, Leake J, et al. Seizures following cardiac surgery: the impact of tranexamic acid and other risk factors. *Can J Anaesth.* 2012;59(1):6–13.

25. Navarro V, Varnous S, Galanaud D, et al. Incidence and risk factors for seizures after heart transplantation. *J Neurol.* 2010;257(4):563–568.

26. Voss LJ, Sleigh JW, Barnard JPM, Kirsch HE. The howling cortex: seizures and general anesthetic drugs. *Anesth Analg.* 2008;107(5):1689–1703.

27. Lowenstein DH, Bleck T, Macdonald RL. It's time to revise the definition of status epilepticus. *Epilepsia.* 1999;40(1):120–122.

28. Chambers HG, Weinstein CH, Mubarak SJ, Wenger DR, Silva PD. The effect of valproic acid on blood loss in patients with cerebral palsy. *J Pediatr Orthopaed.* 1999;19(6):792–795.

6.

POSTTRAUMATIC STRESS DISORDER FOLLOWING SURGERY, INTENSIVE CARE, AND INTRAOPERATIVE AWARENESS

Elliott Karren, Elizabeth L. Whitlock, Thomas L. Rodebaugh, and Michael S. Avidan

INTRODUCTION

Although patients presenting for surgery are frequently concerned about the potential for physical complications, they seldom consider the possible psychological and emotional consequences of their surgery. This is true not simply for patients but also for their caregivers. However, physical and mental disorders are intimately interrelated; traumatic experiences exacerbate medical conditions, and physical disorders precipitate and worsen psychological symptoms.[1] Optimizing postoperative mental health should be an important goal, but achieving that goal requires an improved understanding of the psychological sequelae of surgery. Unfortunately, the multiple factors that predispose patients to postoperative psychiatric morbidity—and the impact of that morbidity—are not currently well understood or appreciated.

Surgery is controlled trauma; stressful events occur in the perioperative period that can lead to traumatic memories. Such memories can form in the operating room during episodes of intraoperative awareness, or postoperatively, commonly in the intensive care unit (ICU). However, even when surgery has gone well and physical recovery is good, patients may form traumatic memories based on what they learn about their surgery and what led to it, perhaps especially if the recovery environment is experienced as unsupportive. Traumatic memories can have long-term psychological sequelae and will lead to symptoms of posttraumatic stress disorder (PTSD) in at least a minority of individuals. In this chapter, we summarize what is known about surgery, ICU experiences, and the development of PTSD. We also specifically explore the relationship between intraoperative awareness and subsequent PTSD.

POSTTRAUMATIC STRESS DISORDER

Unlike disease with obvious physical manifestations, psychiatric diseases have more frequently been stigmatized. Prior to the recognition of PTSD as a psychiatric disorder, sufferers were frequently regarded as neurotic and maladaptive; that is, their personal failings were often seen as the primary reason for their psychological difficulties.[2,3] The experiences of World War II survivors, especially those who suffered extreme trauma in concentration camps, challenged the prevailing dogma.[3] A diagnosis that was similar to PTSD appeared in the *Diagnostic and Statistical Manual of Mental Disorders* (DSM)-I in 1952 under the name "gross stress reaction."[4] Interestingly, this diagnosis was omitted in the DSM-II edition, perhaps because it was published during a period of relative peace.[4] PTSD was recognized as a psychiatric disorder in the DSM-III in 1980,[5] as Vietnam War veterans drew society's (or at least mental health professionals') attention to their suffering.[4] PTSD was defined as a stress disorder that is a final common pathway occurring as a consequence of many different types of stressors, including both combat and civilian stress.[4] For an official diagnosis, patients required an experience that was "outside usual human range" and "markedly distressing to almost anyone." DSM-IV modified the

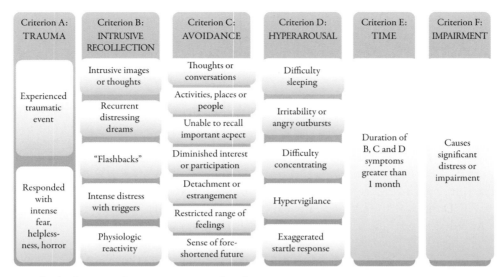

Figure 6.1 DSM-IV criteria for the diagnosis of posttraumatic stress disorder.

diagnosis by dropping the "outside human range" requirement and instead requiring that the experience "involve threatened death, or actual or threatened serious injury, or a threat to the physical integrity of self or others." DSM-IV did not alter any of the characterizing symptoms.

The diagnosis of PTSD is made by six major criteria outlined in DSM-IV. The first major criterion is exposure to the traumatic event, particularly events that involve threatened death or actual or threatened serious injury. Notably in the context of surgery, *exposure* to a traumatic event can occur well after the event itself. For example, an individual who nearly died in a car crash can experience exposure to that traumatic event days or weeks later, after regaining consciousness and learning of the events. In addition to experiencing a traumatic event, patients must also exhibit symptoms across several domains (criteria B, C, D), including *intrusive recollection*, *avoidance*, and *hyperarousal*. Essentially, people with PTSD find themselves thinking about the event despite their best attempts not to, and spend significant periods of time feeling and acting as if the event were very likely to happen again. Lastly, to obtain a formal diagnosis, these symptoms must have lasted longer than 1 month and must also have caused a significant impairment in social or occupational functioning (Criteria E & F) (Figure 6.1). These criteria are still thought by at least some researchers to be too restrictive and are currently under review for the DSM-5.[6] The definition of PTSD raises important questions about the relationship between a stressor, the individual experiencing it, and the characteristic symptoms.[4] PTSD is estimated to have a lifetime prevalence of >6.5% as measured by the National Co-Morbidity Study,[7] and despite the historical combat associations, women are more likely to have PTSD than men (10% vs. 5%).

INTRODUCTION TO INTRAOPERATIVE AWARENESS

General anesthetic agents typically suppress arousal, perception, and memory formation. Unintended intraoperative awareness is recognized to have occurred when patients postoperatively report the memory of sensations that they experienced during the operative period, when they expected to be unaware, and when their clinicians intended them to be unaware. For awareness with recall to occur, a patient must be aroused enough to perceive external stimuli and have an explicit memory formed that they can recall at a postoperative date. Patients who have experienced intraoperative awareness have reported a variety of memories, including tracheal intubation, urine catheter insertion, body positioning, surgical incision, physical restraint, sounds of surgery, voices, music, and feelings of pain, anxiety, and fear.[8] Similar to experiences patients endure in the ICU, these memories can be distressing and traumatic and have been implicated as causing persistent postoperative psychological symptoms, including PTSD.[9,10]

INCIDENCE OF PTSD FOLLOWING ICU STAY, SURGERY, AND INTRAOPERATIVE AWARENESS

ICU STAY AND PTSD

Several psychiatric illnesses, including major depressive disorder, generalized anxiety disorder, and PTSD, are prevalent in ICU survivors. A systematic review by Griffiths et al. found a wide range in PTSD incidence following ICU discharge.[11] Studies in which the diagnosis was made through a structured clinical encounter reported incidences of 4.7% to 52.8%, while those using self-reporting measures had incidences ranging from 1.9% to 63.6%.[11] Studies that involved postsurgical patient populations reported incidences ranging from 1.9% to 52.8%, while those studying medical patient populations had incidences of 9.8 to 63.6%.[11] Overall, there appears to be a high, albeit variable, risk for PTSD following ICU discharge for both medical and surgical ICU patient populations (Figure 6.2). The variability in reported PTSD incidences could be attributable to several factors, including study design, patient populations, the method by which PTSD was diagnosed, and the timing of the post-ICU discharge assessment.[11]

Since the publication of the review by Griffiths et al. there have been several other studies examining the incidence of PTSD following ICU discharge. One study evaluated 313 patients in nine ICU centers, involving both medical and surgical patients.[12] Using a self-reporting tool to measure PTSD symptom severity, the authors reported an incidence of PTSD of 18% at 6 months following ICU discharge. Another large study evaluated 238 patients in five ICUs, also involving both medical and surgical patients. These investigators observed an incidence of PTSD of 9.2% at 3 months following ICU discharge.[13] A further study followed patients from a medical and surgical ICU at the University of Minnesota.[14] This study reported a PTSD incidence of 16.8% (25/149) at 2 months and 15% (12/80) at 6 months following ICU discharge. It is clear that PTSD is an important negative outcome after ICU discharge;

however, it is currently not routinely assessed, and protocols to prevent PTSD during and to treat PTSD following ICU stay have not been developed.

MAJOR SURGERY AND PTSD

It is currently unknown whether surgery contributes to PTSD risk independent of ICU admission; many patients undergoing major surgery are admitted to the ICU, making it difficult to tease out the potential contribution of surgery to psychological symptoms. For example, studies on patients undergoing cardiac surgery, liver transplantation, and major vascular surgery have found PTSD incidences ranging from 5% to 23%.[15-17] In a study by Myhren et al., it was noted that the incidence of PTSD following ICU stay did not differ when the reason for admission was medical, surgical, or trauma related (25% vs. 33% vs. 24% respectively, $p > 0.05$).[18] Griffiths et al. also demonstrated overlap when comparing PTSD incidences in surgical and medical ICU populations (Figure 6.2). Data in relation to psychological sequelae of surgery specifically are sparse and contradictory. In a study at the University of Iowa, 1,420 unselected surgical patients were observed for 3 months after their procedure for postoperative psychiatric disturbances.[19] While overall anxiety decreased after surgery, there was an increase in the subscales for somatic, obsessive-compulsive, and paranoid symptoms. Furthermore, the number of people with severe symptoms in the somatic, obsessive-compulsive, depression, hostility, and paranoia subscales increased after surgery. Although PTSD was not assessed as a discrete end-point, and none of the assessed symptoms are directly indicative of PTSD, we would expect depression, somatization, and paranoia (although notably not *paranoid* or *persecutory delusions*) to all increase when PTSD-related anxiety increases. As such, the observed increases might be explained in part by development of PTSD. This suggests that PTSD might be a relevant postoperative adverse outcome.

INTRAOPERATIVE AWARENESS AND PTSD

Several case reports in the 1960s used the term "traumatic neurosis" to describe the set of postoperative psychiatric symptoms exhibited by patients who became conscious during surgery. It has been difficult to study the link between awareness and PTSD, as intraoperative awareness is relatively uncommon, with an incidence in unselected surgical patients from 0.1% to 0.2%.

Osterman et al. undertook a study to identify PTSD in patients with previous intraoperative awareness.[20] They recruited 16 patients with intraoperative awareness and

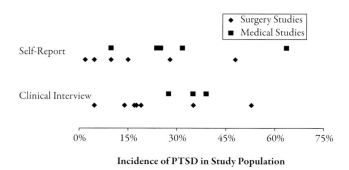

Figure 6.2 Incidence of PTSD following intensive care unit (ICU) stay as reported by Griffiths et al. *Clinical Interview* refers to studies where the PTSD diagnosis was made by formal clinical encounters. *Self-Report* refers to studies where the PTSD diagnosis was made by an empirically supported tool completed by patients. Studies were stratified according to whether they occurred in a medical ICU or medical population (Medical Studies) or a surgical/mixed ICU or specific postsurgical patient populations (Surgical Studies). Data were only reported if a true incidence was available. In studies where multiple incidences were recorded, the first assessed incidence was reported.

compared them with 10 age-matched postsurgical control patients who did not suffer intraoperative awareness. Using a structured clinical interview, they observed that 9 of 16 (56.3%) patients with intraoperative awareness and 0 of 10 controls had PTSD when assessed at a median time of 17 years after the operation. Lennmarken et al. evaluated PTSD in 18 patients who were identified prospectively as having experienced intraoperative awareness from a surgical cohort of 11,785 patients.[9] Two patients could not be reached and one had died; six declined to participate. Nine patients consented to evaluation using a structured clinical encounter; four of the nine (44%) had PTSD at a median of 27 months after their surgery. Ghoneim et al. recently conducted one of the largest studies on risk factors for and consequences of intraoperative awareness by reviewing the published literature over several decades. They examined 271 cases of intraoperative awareness in the literature and found that 22% of the patients had long-term psychological sequelae, including PTSD.[21] They also found that patients who had experienced intraoperative awareness commonly had complaints of sleep disturbances, nightmares, daytime anxiety, and fear of future anesthetics.

A matched cohort study involving patients from the B-Aware trial evaluated the incidence of PTSD in all seven surviving patients that had been prospectively identified to have experienced intraoperative awareness.[10] They were compared with 25 matched control patients who had not experienced intraoperative awareness. Based on rigorous clinical assessment, the investigators found that 5 of 7 patients (71.4%) with intraoperative awareness developed postoperative PTSD, while 3 of 25 (12%) control patients developed postoperative PTSD at a median follow-up period of 5.7 years. One study evaluated the risk of PTSD following intraoperative awareness in children but found that none of the patients (0/7 suffered PTSD) at a median time of 1 year postoperatively, using a self-reporting tool designed specifically for use in a pediatric population.[22]

The studies reviewed here offer widely differing estimates on the precise number of patients who would be expected to develop PTSD, but this is to be expected given small sample sizes and differing assessment methods. More specifically, interview and self-report methods can show considerable differences, from who agrees to complete the report (e.g., interviews may be less convenient) to what is reported when they are completed. Beyond such differences, collectively these studies clearly suggest that PTSD is a common complication of intraoperative awareness for adult surgical patients.

RISK FACTORS FOR PTSD

PATIENT FACTORS

There are several factors that render people more susceptible to developing PTSD. These factors probably increase the likelihood of PTSD following ICU admission, major surgery, or intraoperative awareness. Patients with a psychiatric history, including anxiety or depression, or those who have elevated levels of normal personality characteristics, such as anxiety, pessimism, or, more generally, neuroticism, are at an increased risk of PTSD.[13,18,23] Lower socioeconomic status has also consistently been identified as a predisposing factor for PTSD.[18] These predispositions can be understood as factors that lead people to have an impaired ability to cope with stressful events or emotions. Peritraumatic dissociation is an important risk factor for PTSD, although it is often difficult to assess. Feelings of dissociation surrounding the traumatic event, such as altered sense of time and feeling disconnected from one's body,[24] have been hypothesized to be manifestations of the psychological and physiological response to the trauma, related to feelings of terror and panic that are common responses to such events.[25] Studies have repeatedly found that dissociation during traumatic events is a potent independent predictor of subsequent PTSD.[26]

RISK FACTORS FOR PTSD IN ICU SURVIVORS

With the original restrictive definition of traumas outside the normal range of human experience, PTSD was diagnosed predominantly in those who suffered major trauma in combat situations.[5] With the more expansive definition, other types of stress, including experiences in hospital and surgical settings, were recognized as potential precipitants of PTSD. ICU stay can be associated with many traumatic memories, including those of endotracheal intubation, oropharyngeal suctioning, mechanical ventilation, muscle paralysis, physical restraint, difficulty breathing, and loud alarms. In addition, ICU survivors commonly report delusional memories surrounding their stay. In one study, patients were asked to give detailed descriptions of their ICU stay.[12] Patient responses included memories of being harmed or hurt by nurses and physicians; some patients reported memories of hospital staff trying to kill them. Patients also reported hallucinations during their ICU stay, including the sensation of bugs on their skin (formication) or visitations by deceased family members. In addition to explicit memories, other experiences in the ICU can also potentially be linked to PTSD. These include feelings of discomfort, pain, or confusion, and emotional experiences of intense fear, panic, anxiety, and depression. Further exacerbating the problem, ICU patients are often ill equipped to cope with these experiences. They are often surrounded by strangers, have limited mobility, are unable to communicate, and are subjected to invasive monitoring and procedures. In multiple studies of ICU survivors, patients frequently mention memories in several of these categories. These memories have been implicated as potential precipitants of PTSD.[12] Impairment of sleep cycles, a common problem for ICU patients, probably increases their susceptibility to long-term psychological symptoms.[27] Interestingly, the dose of benzodiazepine sedative medications administered on the ICU has been associated both with increased delirium in the ICU[28] and with increased PTSD following ICU discharge.[29] Although impaired sleep cycles may exacerbate future problems, medically imposed sleep may have similar consequences.

ICU patients are vulnerable as they are often alone in an unfamiliar environment, they are subjected to repeated invasive and painful procedures, and they are often unable to communicate with the hospital staff around them. A study by Granja et al.[12] notes that in reports of ICU memories by survivors, very few are of peaceful and quiet experiences. The majority of descriptions are negative, including feelings of fear, anxiety, and a lack of control. A model of PTSD induction is depicted in Figure 6.3, based on the proposed hypothesis by Granja et al. (Figure 6.3). Central to the model is acute altered sensorium (e.g., delirium, obtundation) induced by some form of insult, whether from trauma, elective major surgery, or an emergency medical condition. The acute alteration in sensorium is worsened during the ICU stay, secondary to potentially modifiable factors such as sedative medications, painful procedures, and sleep disruption. This can lead to modulated memory formation, promoting the formation of delusional memories, which are often traumatic in nature, and can precipitate subsequent PTSD. However, it must be noted that factual memories of ICU experiences can be sufficiently traumatic to engender PTSD.

There is mounting evidence that acute alteration in sensorium during ICU stay favors the formation of PTSD after ICU discharge. Granja et al. found that amnesia of the period before ICU admission was associated with increased odds ratio for PTSD.[12] Additionally, Peris et al. found that a Glasgow Coma Scale (GCS) <9 (indicating unconsciousness) at ICU admission was also associated with increased risk for PTSD.[30] The *duration* of the amnesic period during ICU stay was not found to be associated with PTSD, however.[14] Interestingly, illness severity, as measured by APACHE II or SAPS II scores, were also not associated with an increased incidence of PTSD.[12,13,18,23]

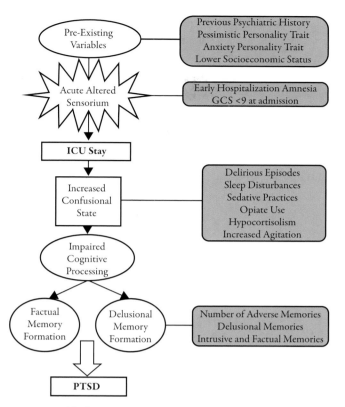

Figure 6.3 Model of posttraumatic stress disorder (PTSD) following intensive care unit (ICU) stay. Briefly, some patients are predisposed to PTSD, through a variety of personality and psychosocial variables that increase emotional reactions to stress or decrease the ability to cope emotionally with stressful events and their consequences. Regardless of predisposition, all patients have some event (trauma, major elective surgery, or emergent medical condition) that leads to altered sensorium, and that incidentally leads to ICU admission. Amnesia concerning the event leading to ICU admission is also known to predispose to PTSD formation. During the ICU stay, patients are subjected to several interventions or experiences that can cause a confused state, including delirious episodes, sleep disturbances, heavy opiate and benzodiazepine use, hypocortisol state, and increased agitation. The sum effect of these variables leads to impaired cognitive processing. Impaired cognitive processing of ICU events facilitates the formation of delusional memories while inhibiting the formation of factual memories. This imbalance has been suggested to promote PTSD. GCS, Glasgow Coma Scale.

Weinert et al. demonstrated that increasing duration of wakefulness on the ICU was associated with PTSD symptoms.[14] Prolonged duration of sedation and opiate use were also found to be also associated with PTSD formation.[13] Physical restraint was associated with an increased risk of PTSD, but this might be reflective of delirium, as patients generally did not remember the restraints.[13]

Curiously, in several studies, patients describe their factual memories of ICU as vague, while delusional memories remained clear, even up to several years after discharge.[13,23] Research findings suggest that delusional memories are associated with an increased risk of PTSD.[12–14,23] An increased number of adverse memories, whether factual or delusional, appear to increase the risk of PTSD.[12,31-34] The literature overall would suggest that it does not matter whether a trauma actually happened in regard to PTSD: what matters is that a person *experiences* an event that he or she perceives as traumatic.

RISK FACTORS FOR PTSD AFTER SURGERY

Although there is strong evidence that intensive care is associated with psychological sequelae, there is limited research into the putative independent contribution of surgery to the subsequent development of PTSD. Plausible modifiable risk factors for PTSD associated with surgery include intraoperative awareness, debilitating postoperative pain, severe postoperative nausea and vomiting, postoperative sleep disturbances, postoperative depression, unexpected medical complications of surgery, unnecessary postoperative tracheal intubation and mechanical ventilation, and avoidable intensive care admission.[16,19] These hypothetical risk factors should be explored in appropriately designed prospective studies. As noted previously, the finding that PTSD appears to be common following ICU admission for both medical and surgical causes (Figure 6.2) does not necessarily imply that surgery does not contribute independently to the risk of PTSD. Patients undergoing major surgery expect to be admitted to ICU, unlike medical patients, who frequently have unexpected ICU admissions for medical emergencies. It might therefore be regarded as surprising that PTSD could be as common following both surgical and medical ICU admissions. It is important to determine the extent to which surgery contributes independently to the risk of persistent psychological symptoms; surgery is a predictable major stressor, and many candidate risk factors are potentially modifiable in the perioperative period.

RISK FACTORS FOR PTSD FOLLOWING INTRAOPERTIVE AWARENESS

It has been convincingly shown that patients who experience intraoperative awareness are at high risk of developing persistent psychological symptoms, including PTSD.[9,10,20] Some patients are more likely to develop PTSD than others, and for them awareness is an important mediator or catalyst that triggers psychological symptoms. The content of the awareness experience is probably an important determinant of risk for persistent psychological symptoms. A variety of memories have been reported, including memories of pain, auditory perceptions, and inability to move.[21] The emotional valence associated with the

memories is also variable but can include fear, hopelessness, and anxiety;[21] such intense negative emotions are thought to promote PTSD.[9] Interestingly, even memories of awareness that are not reported as distressing, such as a feeling of corporal dissociation, have been associated with subsequent PTSD.[20] From a literature review undertaken by Ghoneim et al., memories of an inability to move or of anxiety, panic, or a sense of impending death were associated with later psychological symptoms.[21] Taken together, the data suggest that memories of the awareness experience including a sense of helplessness (inability to move and dissociation from the body) or strongly negative emotional content are the most likely to lead to subsequent PTSD.

PREVENTION OF PTSD

POST-ICU

Certain practices in the ICU can potentially be modified with the goal of preventing acute altered sensorium (e.g., delirium), traumatic memory formation, and perhaps also delusional memory formation. Targeting healthy sleep hygiene, promoting regular contact with family members, alleviating discomfort, and frequently reorienting patients to current time and place might all be helpful interventions (Figure 6.3). The impact of sedation on PTSD is unclear, with recent research suggesting that sedation (e.g., for mechanical ventilation) might not decrease the likelihood of PTSD. Two randomized controlled clinical trials sought to determine whether waking patients while on mechanical ventilation would impact their long-term psychiatric outcomes. One study compared 13 patients who had daily wakening until they were able to follow commands with 19 patients who received routine ICU sedation. Surprisingly, fewer patients in the group that had daily wakening developed PTSD than in the control group (0% vs. 36%, $p = 0.06$).[35] Another study was undertaken in 80 patients in a medical ICU; 48 patients were woken daily and 32 patients received sedation according to routine practice. Patients were assessed for PTSD at 3 and 12 months after ICU discharge.[36] There was no significant difference in PTSD scores at 3 months (14% vs. 10%, $p = 0.59$) and at 12 months (24% vs. 24%, $p = 0.97$). In contrast to the evidence from the operating room, it appears that episodes of awareness in the ICU are not associated with increased risk of subsequent PTSD. The reasons for this surprising finding might be that ICU patients are generally not pharmacologically paralyzed, and they are not undergoing painful surgical procedures. Therefore, unlike the operating room, awareness episodes in the ICU are usually not markedly distressing. Furthermore, during extended ICU stays, it is unrealistic to expect that patients could be prevented from all instances of awareness. Attempting to maintain complete sedation seems, if anything, more likely to lead to delusional memories regarding ICU stay.

Since PTSD could arise from patient difficulty in understanding the delusional and factual memories formed in the ICU, it was hypothesized that if they were offered opportunities to evaluate these memories early on, the incidence of PTSD would decrease.[30] The investigators formed a Clinical Psychology Service (CPS), consisting of three clinical psychologists who were available at all times for consultation in the unit. They provided emotional support and coping strategies to conscious patients with critical illness or major trauma. Their interventions included counseling, stress management strategies, educational services, and coping strategies to ease depression, fear, hopelessness, helplessness, and anxiety. They compared two cohorts of patients, one cohort of 86 patients who had an ICU stay prior to implementation of the CPS (control), with 123 patients who had the service available to them, should they require it. At 12 months postdischarge, the number of patients who were diagnosed with PTSD was higher in the control arm (57%) than the intervention arm (21.1%, $p < 0.001$), and the lack of psychological intervention was associated with a 5-fold increase in risk of PTSD (odds ratio [OR] 5.463, 95% confidence interval [CI] 2.946–10.13). Further research to replicate or refute this intriguing finding is warranted.

Long-term studies of patients with PTSD, including post-ICU patients, have found low serum cortisol levels many years after the traumatic event occurred.[31] High catecholamine and low cortisol concentrations have been suggested to be risk factors for PTSD development.[34] Several studies have examined the potential utility of pharmacologic interventions to prevent PTSD. Therapies that might be promising in this regard include steroids, β-blockers, opiates, ketamine, and α_2 agonists.[33,34,37] Glucocorticoids are thought to enhance episodic memory consolidation while inhibiting the retrieval of emotionally charged autobiographical memories. Administering glucocorticoids in the ICU could potentially enhance consolidation of factual memories and inhibit the recollection of traumatic memories. Steroids and other promising candidate therapies to prevent PTSD should be rigorously assessed in appropriately designed prospective trials.

INTRAOPERATIVE AWARENESS

It is not known how the increased risk for PTSD associated specifically with intraoperative awareness can be mitigated apart from preventing the awareness experience itself. There are several approaches that could potentially decrease the risk and are worth exploring. First, high-risk patients should be counseled about awareness and should be encouraged to report intraoperative awareness, even if at the time they are not distressed by the experience. It might be helpful to identify patient characteristics, such as history of PTSD, anxiety, and depression, which are known risk factors for PTSD. Particular attention could be paid to these patients in the perioperative period, including appropriate sedative medication and targeted postoperative questioning.

Evidence-based approaches to decrease the incidence of intraoperative awareness should adopted, such as protocols based on end tidal volatile anesthetic concentration alerts or processed electroencephalogram alerts.[8,38,39] Minimizing the intraoperative use of muscle relaxants and optimizing intraoperative blockade of nociception (e.g., regional anesthesia or multimodal analgesia) might decrease the distressing experience of awareness if it does occur. An important study showed that morphine given early to combat victims could decrease the incidence of PTSD.[40] Postoperatively, if patients report that they experienced intraoperative awareness, they should be offered therapeutic interventions.

Psychotherapies for PTSD with known effectiveness are generally known as cognitive behavioral therapies and have been shown to decrease symptoms of PTSD and possibly even prevent PTSD.[41] Given the high risk of persistent psychological symptoms following awareness, the best way to prevent postawareness PTSD would be to administer adequate anesthetic and analgesic doses to prevent intraoperative distressing awareness episodes.

GENERAL THERAPY CONSIDERATIONS

PTSD has been thoroughly studied in several nonoperative patient populations, including war veterans, victims of violence, and victims of trauma. Psychotherapy has also been explored, with the most rigorous research focusing on forms of cognitive behavioral therapy, such as prolonged exposure, cognitive processing therapy, and anxiety management training.[42,43] It is essential to note that available evidence suggests that psychotherapy for PTSD is more effective than pharmacologic interventions.[44] As such, psychotherapy should be offered to patients before prescribing medications, which, although helpful for many, are less likely to return people with PTSD to normal functioning.

Multimodal pharmacologic treatment has been suggested for PTSD, including interventions with anxiolytics, β-blockers, steroids, opiates, and selective serotonin reuptake inhibitors (SSRI).[45–47] Of the various candidate drugs, the SSRIs have been most studied and should be used as first-line pharmacologic agents (e.g., if psychotherapy is refused or unavailable).[48] For patients who have undergone major surgery or those who have recently been discharged from an ICU, a reasonable management strategy might be to screen for symptoms of PTSD with a sensitive instrument, such as the Posttraumatic Stress Disorder Checklist-Specific (PCL-S).[49] A structured interview could be offered to those who report symptoms, followed by therapeutic interventions, if indicated. Interventions immediately after a traumatic experience have the potential to work as secondary prevention and to decrease the severity of PTSD symptoms.[47] Overall, however, available studies most strongly support treating PTSD symptoms that arise rather than interventions with people who are not yet experiencing PTSD symptoms in an attempt to prevent it (see http://effectivehealthcare. ahrq.gov/ehc/products/403/1129/Prevention-of-Adult-PTSD_Protocol-Amendment_20120731.pdf)).

CONCLUSION

Posttraumatic stress disorder is a serious and surprisingly common finding in patients who are discharged from an ICU. Although the psychological sequelae of major surgery have not been clarified, patients who experience intraoperative awareness are now known to be at markedly increased risk for developing PTSD. There is clearly a clinical imperative to discover more about postsurgery and post-ICU persistent psychological symptoms and to discover the best approaches to prevent PTSD following these predictable major life events.

CONFLICT OF INTEREST STATEMENT

E.K., E.L.W., T.L.R., and M.S.A. have no conflicts of interest to disclose.

REFERENCES

1. Sledjeski EM, Speisman B, Dierker LC. Does number of lifetime traumas explain the relationship between PTSD and chronic medical conditions? Answers from the National Comorbidity Survey-Replication (NCS-R). *J Behav Med.* 2008;31(4):341–349.
2. Jones E, Wessely S. A paradigm shift in the conceptualization of psychological trauma in the 20th century. *J Anxiety Disord.* 2007;21(2):164–175.
3. Kinzie JD, Goetz RR. A century of controversy surrounding posttraumatic stress stress-spectrum syndromes: the impact on DSM-III and DSM-IV. *J Trauma Stress.* 1996;9(2):159–179.
4. Andreasen NC. Posttraumatic stress disorder: a history and a critique. *Ann N Y Acad Sci.* 2010;1208:67–71.
5. Lasiuk GC, Hegadoren KM. Posttraumatic stress disorder part I: historical development of the concept. *Perspect Psychiatr Care.* 2006;42(1):13–20.
6. Friedman MJ, Resick PA, Bryant RA, Brewin CR. Considering PTSD for DSM-5. *Depress Anxiety.* 2011;28(9):750–769.
7. Elhai JD, Grubaugh AL, Kashdan TB, Frueh BC. Empirical examination of a proposed refinement to DSM-IV posttraumatic stress disorder symptom criteria using the National Comorbidity Survey Replication data. *J Clin Psychiatry.* 2008;69(4):597–602.
8. Avidan MS, Zhang L, Burnside BA, et al. Anesthesia awareness and the bispectral index. *N Engl J Med.* 2008;358(11):1097–1108.
9. Lennmarken C, Bildfors K, Enlund G, Samuelsson P, Sandin R. Victims of awareness. *Acta Anaesthesiol Scand.* 2002;46:(3):229–231.
10. Leslie K, Chan MT, Myles PS, Forbes A, McCulloch TJ. Posttraumatic stress disorder in aware patients from the B-aware trial. *Anesth Analg.* 2010;110(3):823–828.
11. Griffiths J, Fortune G, Barber V, Young JD. The prevalence of post-traumatic stress disorder in survivors of ICU treatment: a systematic review. *Intensive Care Med.* 2007;33(9):1506–1518.
12. Granja C, Gomes E, Amaro A, et al. Understanding posttraumatic stress disorder-related symptoms after critical care: the early illness amnesia hypothesis. *Crit Care Med.* 2008;36(10):2801–2809.
13. Jones C, Backman C, Capuzzo M, Flaatten H, Rylander C, Griffiths RD. Precipitants of post-traumatic stress disorder following intensive care: a hypothesis generating study of diversity in care. *Intensive Care Med.* 2007;33(6):978–985.
14. Weinert CR, Sprenkle M. Post-ICU consequences of patient wakefulness and sedative exposure during mechanical ventilation. *Intensive Care Med.* 2008;34(1):82–90.
15. Liberzon I, Abelson JL, Amdur RL, et al. Increased psychiatric morbidity after abdominal aortic surgery: risk factors for stress-related disorders. *J Vasc Surg.* 2006;43(5):929–934.
16. Rothenhausler H-B, Ehrentraut S, Kapfhammer H-P. Psychiatric and psychosocial outcome of orthotopic liver transplantation. *Psychother Psychosom.* 2002;71(5):13.
17. Schelling G, Richter M, Roozendaal B, et al. Exposure to high stress in the intensive care unit may have negative effects on health-related quality-of-life outcomes after cardiac surgery. *Crit Care Med.* 2003;31(7):1971–1980.
18. Myhren H, Ekeberg O, Toien K, Karlsson S, Stokland O. Posttraumatic stress, anxiety and depression symptoms in patients during the first year post intensive care unit discharge. *Crit Care.* 2010;14(1):R14.
19. Ohara MW, Ghoneim MM, Hinrichs JV, Mehta MP, Wright EJ. Psychological consequences of surgery. *Psychosom Med.* 1989;51(3):356–370.
20. Osterman JE, Hopper J, Heran WJ, Keane TM, van der Kolk BA. Awareness under anesthesia and the development of posttraumatic stress disorder. *Gen Hosp Psychiatry.* 2001;23(4):198–204.
21. Ghoneim MM, Block RI, Haffarnan M, Mathews MJ. Awareness during anesthesia: risk factors, causes and sequelae: a review of reported cases in the literature. *Anesth Analg.* 2009;108(2):527–535.
22. Lopez U, Habre W, Van der Linden M, Iselin-Chaves IA. Intra-operative awareness in children and post-traumatic stress disorder. *Anaesthesia.* 2008;63(5):474–481.
23. Jones C, Griffiths RD, Humphris G, Skirrow PM. Memory, delusions, and the development of acute posttraumatic stress disorder-related symptoms after intensive care. *Crit Care Med.* 2001;29(3):573–580.

24. Marmar CR, Weiss DS, Schlenger WE, et al. Peritraumatic dissociation and posttraumatic stress in male Vietnam theater veterans. *Am J Psychiatry.* 1994;151(6):902–907.

25. Gershuny BS, Cloitre M, Otto MW. Peritraumatic dissociation and PTSD severity: do event-related fears about death and control mediate their relation? *Behav Res Ther.* 2003;41(2):157–166.

26. Ozer EJ, Best SR, Lipsey TL, Weiss DS. Predictors of posttraumatic stress disorder and symptoms in adults: a meta-analysis. *Psychol Bull.* 2003;129(1):52–73.

27. Meerlo P, Sgoifo A, Suchecki D. Restricted and disrupted sleep: effects on autonomic function, neuroendocrine stress systems and stress responsivity. *Sleep Med Rev.* 2008;12(3):197–210.

28. Pandharipande PP, Pun BT, Herr DL, et al. Effect of sedation with dexmedetomidine vs lorazepam on acute brain dysfunction in mechanically ventilated patients: the MENDS randomized controlled trial. *JAMA.* 2007;298(22):2644–2653.

29. Girard TD, Shintani AK, Jackson JC, et al. Risk factors for post-traumatic stress disorder symptoms following critical illness requiring mechanical ventilation: a prospective cohort study. *Crit Care.* 2007;11(1):R28.

30. Peris A, Bonizzoli M, Iozzelli D, et al. Early intra-intensive care unit psychological intervention promotes recovery from post traumatic stress disorders, anxiety and depression symptoms in critically ill patients. *Crit Care.* 2011;15(1):R41.

31. Hauer D, Weis F, Krauseneck T, Vogeser M, Schelling G, Roozendaal B. Traumatic memories, post-traumatic stress disorder and serum cortisol levels in long-term survivors of the acute respiratory distress syndrome. *Brain Res.* 2009;1293:114–120.

32. Sackey PV, Martling CR, Carlsward C, Sundin O, Radell PJ. Short- and long-term follow-up of intensive care unit patients after sedation with isoflurane and midazolam—a pilot study. *Crit Care Med.* 2008;36(3):801–806.

33. Schelling G, Stoll C, Kapfhammer HP, et al. The effect of stress doses of hydrocortisone during septic shock on posttraumatic stress disorder and health-related quality of life in survivors. *Crit Care Med.* 1999;27(12):2678–2683.

34. Schelling G, Kilger E, Roozendaal B, et al. Stress doses of hydrocortisone, traumatic memories, and symptoms of posttraumatic stress disorder in patients after cardiac surgery: a randomized study. *Biol Psychiatry.* 2004;55(6):627–633.

35. Kress JP, Gehlbach B, Lacy M, Pliskin N, Pohlman AS, Hall JB. The long-term psychological effects of daily sedative interruption on critically ill patients. *Am J Respir Crit Care Med.* 2003;168(12):1457–1461.

36. Jackson JC, Girard TD, Gordon SM, et al. Long-term cognitive and psychological outcomes in the awakening and breathing controlled trial. *Am J Respir Crit Care Med.* 2010;182(2):183–191.

37. Weis F, Kilger E, Roozendaal B, et al. Stress doses of hydrocortisone reduce chronic stress symptoms and improve health-related quality of life in high-risk patients after cardiac surgery: a randomized study. *J Thorac Cardiovasc Surg.* 2006;131(2):277–282.

38. Myles PS, Leslie K, McNeil J, Forbes A, Chan MT. Bispectral index monitoring to prevent awareness during anaesthesia: the B-Aware randomised controlled trial. *Lancet.* 2004;363(9423):1757–1763.

39. Avidan MS, Jacobsohn E, Glick D, et al. Prevention of intraoperative awareness in a high-risk surgical population. *N Engl J Med.* 2011;365(7):591–600.

40. Holbrook TL, Galarneau MR, Dye JL, Quinn K, Dougherty AL. Morphine use after combat injury in Iraq and post-traumatic stress disorder. *N Engl J Med.* 2010;362(2):110–117.

41. Kar N. Cognitive behavioral therapy for the treatment of post-traumatic stress disorder: a review. *Neuropsychiatr Dis Treat.* 2011;7:167–181.

42. Mendes DD, Mello MF, Ventura P, Passarela Cde M, Mari Jde J. A systematic review on the effectiveness of cognitive behavioral therapy for posttraumatic stress disorder. *Int J Psychiatry Med.* 2008;38(3):241–259.

43. Bisson J, Andrew M. Psychological treatment of post-traumatic stress disorder (PTSD). *Cochrane Database Syst Rev.* 2007(3):CD003388.

44. Keane TM, Marshall AD, Taft CT. Posttraumatic stress disorder: etiology, epidemiology, and treatment outcome. *Annu Rev Clin Psychol.* 2006;2:161–197.

45. Ipser JC, Stein DJ. Evidence-based pharmacotherapy of post-traumatic stress disorder (PTSD). *Int J Neuropsychopharmacol.* 2012;15(6):825–840.

46. Tarsitani L, De Santis V, Mistretta M, et al. Treatment with beta-blockers and incidence of post-traumatic stress disorder after cardiac surgery: a prospective observational study. *J Cardiothorac Vasc Anesth.* 2012;26(2):265–269.

47. Zohar J, Juven-Wetzler A, Sonnino R, Cwikel-Hamzany S, Balaban E, Cohen H. New insights into secondary prevention in post-traumatic stress disorder. *Dialogues Clin Neurosci.* 2011;13(3):301–309.

48. Stein DJ, Ipser JC, Seedat S. Pharmacotherapy for post traumatic stress disorder (PTSD). *Cochrane Database Syst Rev.* 2006(1):CD002795.

49. McDonald SD, Calhoun PS. The diagnostic accuracy of the PTSD checklist: a critical review. *Clin Psychol Rev.* 2010;30(8):976–987.

PART II

SPINAL CORD

7.

CERVICAL SPINE INJURY

Mazen A. Maktabi

INTRODUCTION TO THE CLINICAL PROBLEM

Perioperative injuries of the cervical spinal cord are rare but are devastating to the patient when they occur. In some cases, the cause of the injury is clear, and in others it is not entirely clear. There is pervasive thinking among anesthesia providers and other health care professionals that perioperative airway management is linked to postoperative spinal cord injury, despite the fact that the number of clinical reports attributing this complication to airway management is small.[1] The clinician is faced with one of two possible clinical scenarios:

1. The patient has known cervical spine risk factors, or the surgery is associated with cervical spinal cord injury risks that are clear. This knowledge in turn triggers precautions and alterations in the routine clinical management to prevent postoperative injury from taking place.

2. The complication (postoperative cervical spinal cord injury) occurs in a patient with no known or well-understood risk factors from the medical history and record.

Thus, the clinical questions are the following: First, are we able to prevent postoperative cervical spinal cord injuries in patient with known risk factors or when the surgery

(such cervical spine surgery) adds risk to the patient? Second, when the surgery does not involve the cervical spine, can we identify the patient at risk for postoperative cervical spine injury and perhaps implement measures to prevent the occurrence of such injuries?

INCIDENCE, PREVALENCE, AND OUTCOMES

Patients who are clearly at risk for postoperative cervical spine injury are those undergoing cervical spine surgeries for degenerative cervical spine disease. On the basis of the Nationwide Inpatient Sample database, Patil et al. reported that the number of cervical surgeries for degenerative cervical spine in the database increased from 53,810 in 1990 to 112,400 in 2000.[2] The surgeries are increasingly performed in older patients, patients with associated systemic illnesses, women, and underrepresented minorities. Surgeries to treat degenerative spine disease vastly outnumber those for traumatic injuries or cervical spine instabilities—90% versus 5–7%.[1] Cervical spondylotic myelopathy (CSM) is a degenerative spine disorder associated with increasing compression of the cervical neural tissues (spinal cord or nerve roots or both) and is the most frequent reason for surgical interventions. Dysphagia, which is thought to be a surgically related neurologic complication of such interventions, appears to be more common with combined anterior–posterior approaches (21.1%) as opposed to exclusively anterior

(2.3%) or exclusively posterior cervical surgeries (0.9%).[3] Other neurologic complications include C5 radiculopathy (1.7–8.5%).[3]

When high-risk surgeries (such as spine and vascular) are excluded, perioperative spinal cord injury (SCI) is rare. SCI was attributed to intubation in only 10 reports;[1] 9 cases of SCI with consequent quadriparesis have been reported following posterior fossa surgery predominantly in the sitting position but also in the prone position.[1,4–7] Hitselberger and House[4] reported five cases of midcervical quadriplegia after acoustic tumor resection performed with the patient in the sitting position. The scarcity of reports of this complication suggests that it is uncommon, but one has to consider the possibility that not all such cases are reported.

Central cord syndrome (CSS) is another manifestation of cervical spinal cord injury that has been associated with endotracheal intubation, intraoperative positioning, and surgery. The neuroanatomic basis of this injury is damage to the lateral corticospinal tracts resulting in motor weakness and sensory deficits, which are more pronounced in the upper extremities than in the lower limbs. Patients with this injury may partially recover some of the deficits. CCS is usually produced as a result of high-velocity hyperextension, but it has been also described following low-velocity hyperextension as with direct laryngoscopy,[8] cervical spine surgery in the sitting position, and cervical spine (C3–C7) posterior decompression.[9] Decreased spinal cord perfusion due to neck flexion and the sitting position appears to have played a role in the development of central cord syndrome in the sitting position. CSS has been reported by several authors in a variety of intraoperative settings.

SCI has been also reported to occur 8 days after a cervical epidural administration of steroid in one patient without any risk factors. There are also scattered reports of postoperative neurologic deficits attributed to antlantoaxial dislocations in patients afflicted with Down and Grisel syndromes.

RISK FACTORS

The unambiguous and most common risk factor for postoperative cervical spine injury is cervical spine surgery. Following cervical laminectomy, the incidence of spinal cord injury varies from 0% to 3%, and injury to nerve roots may be closer to 15%. In addition, recent reports suggest that perioperative complications (including cervical spine complications) of surgery for cervical myelopathy were associated with increased age, combined anteroposterior cervical spine surgeries, increased operative time, and increased blood loss.[3]

Cervical spine myelopathy is a major pre-existing risk factor for development of postoperative cervical neurologic injury in noncervical spine surgery. This is a condition that results from sagittal narrowing of the spinal canal, leading to compression of the spinal cord. Excluding, tumors, trauma, and hematomas, the cause of narrowing may be congenital or acquired through degenerative spine disease. The latter condition is common with compression of neural elements in patients older than 70 years of age, although by the age of 55 up to 30% of patients may have compression of the cervical spinal cord (myelopathy) and nerve roots (radiculopathy). The spinal canal may be narrowed by bulging and/or herniated intervertebral discs, osteophytes, hypertrophied posterior longitudinal ligament (particularly in Japanese individuals), and thickened hypertrophied ligamentum flavum. Intervertebral foramina of the cervical spine may also be narrowed by degenerative disease. These lesions develop slowly, occupy space in the spinal canal, and exert chronic compression on the spinal cord (which is normally a very resilient anatomic structure). Impingement on the spinal canal leaves less space between the dura mater and the spinal cord and may thus compromise the cord's blood supply, rendering it vulnerable to further compression. As encroachment increases with time, the spinal cord adopts the changing volumetric and deformed shape as the space diminishes until there is no more room to spare. This slowly developing pathology is frequently associated with no or only subtly discernable clinical symptoms or signs. At the stage of critical compression, any acutely added stretch of the neural tissues with hyperextension (such as during sudden movements, direct laryngoscopy, or positioning) will rapidly increase the compression to the point of producing one or all of the following: acute ischemia, compression injury, tissue edema, hemorrhage, and clinical neurologic deficit. Therefore, pre-existing cervical spondylosis and spinal stenosis of degenerative spine disease are predisposing risk factors for occurrence of postoperative CSS or quadriplegia or quadiparesis. Another key point is that some patients may be free of neurologic symptoms before the "tipping point event" (accident) despite the presence of an acquired or congenital spinal stenosis.[11–13] In other patients, the causative event may be so minor that they cannot even pinpoint its occurrence.

Cervical neural injuries have been reported to occur following emergent intubations that involve cardiovascular resuscitation of patients. Emergent intubations may occur under duress, suboptimal conditions of positioning and airway equipment, poor hemodynamic status, and time pressure. Undue force is not infrequently necessary under these conditions to obtain an adequate view of the glottis in order to insert the endotracheal tube. However, in patients with advanced degenerative cervical spine disease and critical compression of neural tissues, a routine and uncomplicated intubation (that produces what we normally expect as far as neck extension is concerned) may result in profound quadriparesis. There are reports of patients with advanced degenerative changes in which acute compression of neural tissue and severe neurologic injury occurred without any concomitant dislocations or fractures of the bony elements of the neck. Narrowing of the spinal canal developmentally, by a thickened and ossified posterior longitudinal ligament, or cervical spondylosis[14–16] has been associated with spinal cord compressions, infarctions, or injuries that occurred following minor low-velocity trauma without associated fractures of bony elements or dislocations of the cervical spine.

In addition to neurologic injury brought about by extension of the cervical spine for oral endotracheal intubation, a similar mechanism of injury resulting in postoperative quadriparesis is prolonged neck extension, such as in parathyroidectomies in patients with end-stage renal disease on long-term hemodialysis. These patients may develop a condition known as destructive spondyloarthropathy (DSA).[17,18] This condition consists of two components. The first involves inflammation of the spinal joints and collapse of the intervertebral disc, resulting in abnormal spine motion and neural compression. The second element of DSA is extensive amyloid deposition extradurally that produces spinal stenosis. Both elements of DSA make the cervical spinal cord and cervical nerve roots prone to compression and neurapraxia when the neck is extended for the duration of the surgery.

Ankylosing spondylitis (AS) is a chronic inflammatory illness affecting primarily the sacroiliac joints and the spine. This disorder is characterized by a gradual progressive inflammatory process that eventually leads to generalized stiffness of the spine (radiographically, the "bamboo spine"). Its prevalence is 0.1–1.4%, and men are affected more than women. Clinically, the disease is detectable in patients at the age of 20 to 30 years.[19] In patients with advanced stages of this disorder, the spine is prone to fractures following low-energy impacts, such as riding a vehicle on bumpy terrain, simple falls into a chair, and falling from the standing or sitting positions. Some patients do not remember any event that led to the fracture.[20] Fractures affect mostly the cervical spine at the junctions of the fused and mobile segments. The cervical spine is more vulnerable than the other parts of the spine because of its increased mobility, small vertebral bodies, oblique articular facets, and mobility of the heavy skull on the cervical spine. Because of the increased risk of fractures in ankylosed spines, it has been recommended that cervical spine fractures be ruled out in trauma patients with ankylosed segments. The challenge facing the clinician in trauma cases presenting with pre-existing AS is that occult fractures of the cervical spine may be present following low-energy injuries. Such fractures are not detectable with the usual imaging studies (plain X-rays, computed tomography [CT] scans, magnetic resonance imaging [MRI] studies). High-definition multidetector CT scanning is more reliable in detecting occult fractures.[21] Thus, in patients with AS, a high index of suspicion is important regarding occult cervical fractures if there is cervical spinal pain after minor or low-impact trauma.[20,22] In addition to vertebral and sacroiliac joints, AS commonly affects temporomandibular and laryngeal joints. This can cause difficulty of mouth opening (during laryngoscopy) and possibly laryngeal joint injuries (during intubation).[20] Systemic manifestations of the disease include peripheral arthritis, iritis, carditis, pulmonary involvement, colitis, and osteoporosis.

Extreme flexion of the neck for an extended period of time is frequently encountered in posterior fossa and cervical spine surgeries to facilitate surgical exposure. Several reports of postoperative quadriparesis[4–6] suggested that the sitting position was a risk factor predisposing to this complication. The combination of neck flexion, the sitting position, and periods of hypotension of variable duration were noted in the reported cases. Several mechanisms of injury have been suggested in this context: compromise of blood supply to the cervical cord by impingement due to arthritic changes and intervertebral bulging discs; reduction of perfusion brought about by the sitting position with or without associated hypotension; stretching of the spinal cord and its blood vessels by extreme flexion; and engorgement of the cervical epidural venous plexus, thus compressing the spinal cord and increasing cerebrospinal fluid (CSF) pressure.[23] The negative impact of the sitting position on perfusion of the spinal cord in the presence of cervical stenosis was emphasized in a clinical report of a patient sustaining postoperative quadriparesis following shoulder surgery in the sitting position.[24] Spinal cord infarction and quadriplegia are also complications of surgery of the posterior fossa in the prone position.[7] As with the sitting position, extended hyperflexion, overstretching of the spinal cord, and compromise of spinal cord blood flow were thought to be contributing factors.

Down syndrome, a common chromosomal abnormality with an incidence of 1 in 1000 live births, is of particular interest to the anesthesiologist because of the associated cardiac, respiratory, and craniospinal abnormalities (15% of patients) that result in atlanto-occipital and/or atlantoaxial instabilities (the latter being more common). It is intuitively obvious to attribute postoperative neurologic injuries in these patients to neck extension during direct laryngoscopy. However, only two cases have been reported that possibly related postoperative neurologic injuries to laryngoscopy and intubation.[25] Three reports related postoperative injury to rotational positioning of the head during head and neck surgery and atrial septal defect repair.[25] Clearly, patients with this inherited disorder are at risk for neurologic injury at the level of the cervical spine if they have craniocervical instability.

Given the frequency of this disorder, how do we identify those at risk? It is important to perform a careful preoperative evaluation to detect symptomatic patients—that is, those with cervical myelopathy. A targeted evaluation of neurologic abnormalities can be conducted through detailed history-taking and a physical examination. The following should be ruled out prior to elective surgery: new behavior changes, worsening of motor abilities, worsening of bowel or bladder functions, pain in the neck or head, difficulty moving the head, syncope or dizziness, and abnormalities in ambulation. Positive findings for any of these criteria constitute grounds for postponement of elective surgery and referral to a specialist to rule out cervical spine instabilities. If the history and physical examination are negative, imaging of the cervical spine may be considered. Ossification of the cervical spine is usually complete by the age of 3 years. Therefore, obtaining plain neck radiographs between the ages of 3 and 5 years would be useful to better identify the bony anatomy. A neck radiograph should be taken if there is prior evidence of bony abnormality, a new clinical neurologic finding by history or physical examination, and if the planned surgery involves movement of the head and neck to anything beyond the neutral position. Communication with the surgical team is of paramount importance preoperatively and during the surgical huddle, regarding intraoperative manipulations, rotational movement, and positioning of the head and neck (especially in otolaryngologic surgeries). If the anesthesiologist is presented with a patient with Down syndrome for an emergency procedure and there is no information on the status of cervical spine stability or anatomy, he or she is faced with difficult decisions regarding the method of securing the airway. Every effort should be made to perform endotracheal intubation using a method that minimizes cervical spine motion (e.g., fiberoptic intubation, intubation through a laryngeal mask airway, lightwand, Bullard™ laryngoscope). There is no consensus among clinical anesthesiologists on how to best manage patients with Down syndrome, and a wide spectrum of practices is encountered. Some require

plain lateral radiographs in flexion and extension before every surgical procedure, while others require imaging only prior to certain surgical procedures. The American Academy of Pediatrics suggests imaging between the ages of 3 and 5 years. Our recommendation to the clinician is to look for new symptoms or signs of cervical myelopathy in the child and to follow that lead with the help of a specialist to rule out cervical spine instability. Other conditions that may be associated with atlantoaxial subluxation are summarized in Table 7.1.

Rheumatoid arthritis (RA), an autoimmune inflammatory disorder that affects synovial joints, systemic organs, and the cervical spine, is the most common chronic inflammatory arthritis and affects about 1% of the adult population. Women (ages 30–50 years) are affected three times more than men. RA often involves the cervical spine (25% to 86% of patients) and is the most common inflammatory disorder affecting the cervical spine.[26] In some patients the disease progresses slowly in a chronic fashion, and in others it progresses rapidly in an aggressive fashion. The occipitocervical junction develops complications in 30% to 50% of patients who suffer from the disease for more than 7 years, and atlantoaxial instabilities with cord compression occur in 2.5% of patients who have the disorder for greater than 14 years.[26] Unlike the remainder of the vertebral column, the occiput-C1 and atlantoaxial joints have only synovial joints without intervertebral discs and thus have less protection than what the discs provide to the remainder of the intervertebral joints. The transverse ligament can become lax, which in advanced cases may result in ligamentous rupture and partial instability of C1–C2 joint (4–5 mm of

Table 7.1 CONDITIONS ASSOCIATED WITH ATLANTOAXIAL SUBLAXATION

Congenital

Down syndrome

Odontoid anomalies

Mucopolysaccharaidosis

Acquired

Rheumatoid arthritis

Stills disease

Ankylosing spondylitis

Psoriatic arthritis

Enteropathic arthritis: Crohn's disease and ulcerative colitis

Reiters syndrome

Trauma: odontoid fractures and ligamentous disruptions

Reproduced with permission from Crosby ET, Lui A. The adult cervical spine implications for airway management. *Can J Anaesth.* 1990;37(1):77–93.[33]

anterior displacement). With involvement of the secondary ligaments that hold the odontoid process in place (alar and apical ligaments), complete subluxation of C1 over C2 may occur. Eventually, the disease process affects the odontoid process, which may turn into a mass of inflammatory tissue; the odontoid process may be deformed and compress the spinal cord or protrude cranially through the foramen magnum and compress the brainstem. Atlantoaxial subluxation is the most common deformity produced by RA and can be anterior, posterior, cranial (with settling and vertical subluxation), lateral/rotatory, subaxial (C2 and below), or a combination of any of these types.[27] Along with these subluxations, various degrees of compression of the neuraxis take place.

With long-standing RA, instability and neural compression occur in a substantial portion of patients. Intuitively, one expects to also encounter a significant number of reports of neurologic injury as a result of direct laryngoscopy and intubation given the frequency of instability of the cervical spine. In reality, there are only eight individual case reports of spinal cord injury due to cervical spine instability of all types[1] that are related to endotracheal intubation; and only one of these is linked to RA.[28] There are two possible reasons for this rare incidence of spinal cord injury. The first is that the occurrence of spinal cord injury with RA during laryngoscopy and intubation is truly low and rare. The second possibility is that this type of injury is underreported.

The question of whether to obtain neck radiographs before conducting elective surgeries is still contentious and there is no consensus or published recommendations in that regard. If a patient presents with a history of RA and no neck plain radiographs are available, there would clearly be a need to obtain lateral plain radiographs in flexion and extension to determine the degree of instability. Other indications for obtaining plain radiographs of the neck are neck pain, new onset of weakness and/or radicular symptoms, and the presence of erosive and aggressive progression of the disease. Knowing the status of cervical spine stability is important for both airway management and neck positioning during the surgical procedure as well as to determine which type of motion would be deleterious to a particular patient affected with RA (flexion, extension, or rotation). The various pros and cons regarding this topic are summarized in Table 7.2.[27]

PREVENTIVE STRATEGIES, TREATMENT, CURRENT GUIDELINES OR RECOMMENDATIONS

What can the clinician do when faced with a patient with *known* cervical spine instability? The answer varies, depending on whether the surgery is elective or emergent. A thorough medical history and physical examination are essential. Review of imaging information is key in determining the best airway management plan of the patient with a known cervical spine instability. Direct laryngoscopy and intubation are not contraindicated in all patients with atlanto-occipital abnormalities. On occasion, in some patients with deformed odontoid processes protruding into the brainstem or the spinal cord, neck extension relieves this impingement, and direct laryngoscopy would be advantageous (in the absence of ligaments laxity). In contrast, in cases of advanced RA with erosion of the odontoid process,

Table 7.2 ARGUMENTS FOR AND AGAINST CERVICAL RADIOGRAPHS IN RHEUMATOID ARTHRITIS

ARGUMENTS FOR RADIOGRAPHS	ARGUMENTS AGAINST RADIOGRAPHS
Asymptomatic subluxation is common.	There is a decline in the incidence and severity of cervical instability and associated neurologic involvement in recent years.
Flexion/extension radiographs are good predictors of difficult direct laryngoscopy.	No difference in anesthetic management of patients with or without cervical instability. There are no reported neurologic complications.
There is no standard "safe" head position—the "protrusion position" may reduce atlantodental interval in anterior AAS but may worsen posterior subluxation.	A total of 77 rheumatoid patients underwent 132 operations. A third of the preoperative cervical spine X-rays were inadequate or of limited diagnostic value.
Proven instability on radiographs alters anesthetic management by reducing neck manipulation.	Serial cervical radiographs over the past 2 years in 14 patients with craniocervical instability showed no progression.
The incidence of AAS progresses over time, rising 4-fold after the third decade. Serial X-rays may show disease progression regardless of findings on previous films.	Obtaining radiographs may delay surgery and expose patients to unnecessary radiation and not alter management.

AAS, atlantoaxial subluxation.
Adapted with permission from Samanta R, Shoukrey K, Griffiths R. Rheumatoid arthritis and anaesthesia. *Anaesthesia.* 2011;66(12):1146–1159.[27]

ligamentous rupture, and spine displacements, one should follow an airway management method that prevents worsening of displacement of vertebral bodies or impingement on neural tissues. In continuous lateral fluoroscopic cadaver studies performed on posteriorly destabilized third cervical (C3) vertebra, Brimacombe et al.[29] provided evidence that "in the cadaver model of a destabilized third cervical vertebrae, significant displacement of the injured segment occurs during airway management with the face mask, laryngoscope-guided oral intubation, the esophageal tracheal Combitube (Kendall-Sheridan, Neustadt, Germany), the intubating and standard laryngeal mask airway, but not with fiberscope-guided nasal intubation. For cervical motion and the techniques tested, the safest airway technique with this injury is fiberscope-guided nasotracheal intubation. Laryngeal mask devices are preferable to the esophageal tracheal Combitube." Fluoroscopy during airway management has also been successfully used in unstable RA patients. A word of caution is warranted, however: despite the use of safe methods during intubation of patients with suspected or documented cervical spine instability, postoperative cervical spinal cord damage has still occurred.[1] This suggests that there are remaining factors that we do not yet understand or know about that contribute to the occurrence of perioperative spinal cord injury.

In patients with known cervical spine myelopathy, every effort should be made intraoperatively to preserve perfusion of the spinal cord through blood pressure maintenance or avoidance of positioning that promotes compression and impairs blood supply of neural tissue (excessive neck flexion, stretching of shoulders, positions that impair venous drainage of the head and neck). Cervical spine myelopathy is not always easy to detect clinically in a previously undiagnosed patient, and only a portion of patients with lumbar spine myelopathy suffer from cervical spine myelopathy as well. Eighteen clinically used tests were evaluated for their ability to detect cervical spine myelopathy, and all were found to have high levels of specificity but low levels of sensitivity, suggesting that they are ineffective screening tools.[30]

Advanced Trauma Life Support guidelines state that manual in-line stabilization (MILS) should be used during direct laryngoscopy and intubation in patients with suspected unstable cervical spine. Its purported advantage is prevention of motion of the unstable cervical spine during direct laryngoscopy. Available evidence does not support this contention. Application of MILS worsens glottic views during intubation, forcing laryngoscopists to apply more upward force in an effort to improve the view. Direct laryngoscopy transmits forces to the cervical spine (with and without MILS). The upward force is transmitted to the cervical spine, which in turn may produce further displacements, thus mitigating the purported benefits of MILS.[31,32] When the clinician is faced with a situation where the airway has to be secured promptly in order to save the life of a patient, any method that safely achieves that purpose (given the clinical circumstances and the best available clinical skills) should be used. This judgment should be left to the clinician on site.

CONCLUSION

Perioperative cervical spine complications of anesthetic care are rare but devastating events. In patients with known cervical spine instability, techniques of intubation that minimize cervical spine motion ought to be used in elective cases. Current evidence suggests that in some patients these techniques, as well as spine immobilization procedures, do not always prevent postoperative neurologic damage. Circumstances of emergency intubations may not allow use of these techniques; clinicians should thus use their judgment as to what is best for their patients.

CONFLICT OF INTEREST STATEMENT

M.A.M. has no conflicts of interest to disclose.

REFERENCES

1. Hindman BJ, Palacek JP, Posner KL, et al. Cervical spinal cord, root, and bony spine injuries. A closed claim analysis. *Anesthesiology*. 2011;114(4):782–795.
2. Patil PG, Turner DA, Pietrobon R. National trends in surgical procedures for degenerative cervical spine disease: 1990–2000. *Neurosurgery*. 2005;57(4):753–758; discussion 753–758.
3. Fehlings MG, Smith JS, Kopjar B, et al. Perioperative and delayed complications associated with the surgical treatment of cervical spondylotic myelopathy based on 302 patients from the AO Spine North America Cervical Spondylotic Myelopathy Study. *J Neurosurg Spine*. 2012;16(5):425–432.
4. Hitselberger WE, House WF. A warning regarding the sitting position for acoustic tumor surgery. *Arch Otolaryngol*. 1980;106:69.
5. Matjasko J, Petrozza P, Cohen M, Steinberg P. Anesthesia and surgery in the seated position: analysis of 554 cases. *Neurosurgery*. 1985;17:695–702.
6. Morandi X, Riffaud L, Amlashi SF, Brassier G. Extensive spinal cord infarction after posterior fossa surgery in the sitting position: case report. *Neurosurgery*. 2004;54(6):1512–1515.
7. Rau CS, Liang CL, Lui CC, Lee TC, Lu K. Quadriplegia in a patient who underwent posterior fossa surgery in the prone position. Case report. *J Neurosurg*. 2002;96(1 Suppl):101–103.
8. Buchowski JM, Kebaish KM, Suk KS, Kostuik JP. Central cord syndrome after total hip arthroplasty: a patient report. *Spine* (Phila Pa 1976). 2005;30(4):E103–E105. Erratum in 2005;30(7):845.

9. Smith PN, Balzer JR, Khan MH, et al. Intraoperative somatosensory evoked potential monitoring during anterior cervical discectomy and fusion in nonmyelopathic patients—a review of 1,039 cases. *Spine J.* 2007;7:83–87.

10. Khan MH, Smith PN, Balzer JR, et al. Intraoperative somatosensory evoked potential monitoring during cervical spine corpectomy surgery: experience with 508 cases. *Spine* 2006;31:E105–E113.

11. Firooznia H, Ahn JH, Rafii M, Ragnarsson KT. Sudden quadriplegia after a minor trauma. The role of preexisting spinal stenosis. *Surg Neurol.* 1985;23(2):165–168.

12. Kudo T, Sato Y, Kowatari K, Nitobe T, Hirota K. Postoperative transient tetraplegia in two patients caused by cervical spondylotic myelopathy. *Anaesthesia.* 2011;66(3):213–216.

13. Young IA, Burns SP, Little JW. Sudden onset of cervical spondylotic myelopathy during sleep: a case report. *Arch Phys Med Rehabil.* 2002;83(3):427–429.

14. Bhatoe HS Spinal cord injury. *J Neurosurg.* 2001;94(2 Suppl):339–340.

15. Koyanagi I, Iwasaki Y, Hida K, Imamura H, Fujimoto S, Akino M. Acute cervical cord injury associated with ossification of the posterior longitudinal ligament *Neurosurgery.* 200353(4):887–891; discussion 891–892.

16. Onishi E, Sakamoto A, Murata S, Matsushita M. Risk factors for acute cervical spinal cord injury associated with ossification of the posterior longitudinal ligament. *Spine* (Phila Pa 1976). 2012;37(8):660–666.

17. Nokura K, Koga H, Yamamoto H, et al. Dialysis-related spinal canal stenosis: a clinicopathological study on amyloid deposition and its AGE modification. *J Neurol Sci.* 2000;178(2):114–123.

18. Ohashi K, Hara M, Kawai R, et al. Cervical discs are most susceptible to beta 2-microglobulin amyloid deposition in the vertebral column. *Kidney Int.* 1992;41(6):1646–1652.

19. Braun J, Sieper J. Ankylosing spondylitis. *Lancet.* 2007;369 (9570):1379–1390.

20. Salathé M, Jöhr M. Unsuspected cervical fractures: a common problem in ankylosing spondylitis. *Anesthesiology.* 1989;70(5):869–870.

21. Elgafy H, Bransford RJ, Chapman JR. Epidural hematoma associated with occult fracture in ankylosing spondylitis patient: a case report and review of the literature. *J Spinal Disord Tech.* 2011;24(7):469–473.

22. Harrop JS, Sharan A, Anderson G, et al. Failure of standard imaging to detect a cervical fracture in a patient with ankylosing spondylitis. *Spine* (Phila Pa 1976). 2005;30(14):E417–E419.

23. Kitahara Y, Iida H, Tachibana S. Effect of spinal cord stretching due to head flexion on intramedullary pressure. *Neurol Med Chir* (Tokyo). 1995;35(5):285–288.

24. Lewandrowski KU, McLain RF, Lieberman I, Orr D. Cord and cauda equina injury complicating elective orthopedic surgery. *Spine* (Phila Pa 1976). 2006;31(9):1056–1059.

25. Hata T, Todd MM. Cervical spine considerations when anesthetizing patients with Down syndrome. *Anesthesiology.* 2005;102(3):680–685.

26. Wasserman BR, Moskovich R, Razi AE. Rheumatoid arthritis of the cervical spine-clinical considerations. *Bull NYU Hosp Jt Dis.* 2011;69(2):136–148.

27. Samanta R, Shoukrey K, Griffiths R. Rheumatoid arthritis and anaesthesia. *Anaesthesia.* 2011;66(12):1146–1159.

28. Yaszemski MJ, Shepler TR. Sudden death from cord compression associated with atlanto-axial instability in rheumatoid arthritis. A case report. *Spine* 1990;15:338–341.

29. Brimacombe J, Keller C, Künzel KH, Gaber O, Boehler M, Pühringer F. Cervical spine motion during airway management: a cinefluoroscopic study of the posteriorly destabilized third cervical vertebrae in human cadavers. *Anesth Analg.* 2000;91(5):1274–1278.

30. Cook CE, Wilhelm M, Cook AE, Petrosino C, Isaacs R. Clinical tests for screening and diagnosis of cervical spine myelopathy: a systematic review. *J Manipulative Physiol Ther.* 2011;34(8):539–546.

31. LeGrand SA, Hindman BJ, Dexter F, Weeks JB, Todd MM. Craniocervical motion during direct laryngoscopy and orotracheal intubation with the Macintosh and Miller Blades. An in vivo cinefluoroscopic study. *Anesthesiology* 2007;107:884–891.

32. Santoni BG, Hindman BJ, Puttlitz CM, et al. Manual in-line stabilization increases pressures applied by the laryngoscope blade during direct laryngoscopy and orotracheal intubation. *Anesthesiology.* 2009;110(1):24–31.

33. Crosby ET, Lui A. The adult cervical spine implications for airway management. *Can J Anaesth.* 1990;37(1):77–93.

8.

SPINAL CORD INJURY AND PROTECTION

Rehan Siddiqui and Rae M. Allain

INTRODUCTION TO THE CLINICAL PROBLEM

Postoperative paraplegia or paraparesis due to spinal cord injury (SCI) is a devastating complication that continues to pose a major risk to patients undergoing surgery of the thoracic and thoracoabdominal aorta. In recent decades, significant work has contributed to improved descriptions of the epidemiology and risks factors for this complication, better understanding of the mechanism of injury, and identification of measures to prevent or reduce the risk.

INCIDENCE, PREVALENCE, AND OUTCOMES

Studies of the prevalence of thoracic aortic disease (aneurysms and/or dissections) over time demonstrate an increasing trend, likely due to improved diagnostic techniques and enhanced population databases. Estimates from a single-nation, population-based study[1] revealed an incidence of thoracic aortic disease of 9 and 16 per 100,000 person years, in women and men, respectively, in 2002. Surgeries on the thoracic aorta occurred at a rate of 3 per 100,000 person years in women and 6 per 100,000 person years in men, with the median age at operation of 63 years. Thirty-day mortality rates are significant and affected by etiology of disease (22% for aortic dissection, 8% for non-

ruptured aneurysm) and presence of aortic rupture (35% if ruptured and 7.6% if not ruptured).

The risk for spinal cord ischemia or infarction during open repair of thoracoabdominal aortic aneurysms (TAA) ranges from approximately 3% to 28%, with lower rates (<10%) reported from high-volume centers and a higher incidence (25% or greater) with emergency operation.[2,3] Endovascular repair of thoracic aortic disease is associated with a lower risk of spinal cord ischemia, approximately 3–12%, although risk may be higher in specific patient populations, including those who have undergone prior abdominal aortic aneurysm repair or those requiring more extensive aortic coverage for treatment.[4,5]

In addition to aneurysm and dissection, other pathologic processes may affect the descending thoracic aorta, including intramural hematoma, penetrating atherosclerotic ulcer, and aortic transection. Each may be associated with paraplegia or paraparesis depending on the location and extent of lesion.

The outcomes of patients who suffer SCI during open TAA surgery is poor. Coselli et al.[6] showed an operative mortality rate approaching 50%, a 10-fold higher rate compared to patients without paralysis. Conrad et al.[7] studied 64 patients with SCI after open or endovascular TAA repair, finding a perioperative mortality of 23% compared to 8% in the uninjured patients. Patients with a more severe motor deficit fared worse in terms of in-hospital complications, ambulatory recovery, and death. All 64 patients with SCI suffered one or more additional significant complications; most common were pulmonary complications, including prolonged respiratory failure and pneumonia. Average intensive care unit (ICU) and hospital length of stay of the cohort was 9 and 25 days, respectively. At 2 years follow-up, no patient with a flaccid paralysis was ambulatory, whereas 73% of patients presenting with <50% motor function had ambulatory recovery. This percentage rose to 100% for patients whose initial motor function was >50% at time of SCI presentation. (The definition of *ambulatory* in this study included patients who walked independently and those who required assistive devices such as canes or walkers). Five-year mortality was 75% with SCI and 49% without. Notably, all of the long-term mortality in the SCI group was accounted for by the patients with flaccid paralysis. Keith et al.[4] examined outcomes of 239 patients who underwent thoracic endovascular aortic repair (TEVAR), finding a 6% SCI rate. The 1-year mortality rate of patients who had SCI was significantly higher (56%) than that for uninjured patients (20%), representing an odds ratio of death within a year of 3.0 for the cord-injured patients.

The etiology of spinal cord ischemia and infarction during thoracic and thoracoabdominal aortic surgery (TA/TAA) appears multifactorial, but disruption of the vascular supply to the spinal cord is a key component. The normal anatomy of the spinal cord vascular supply is shown in Figures 8.1 and 8.2. As seen in Figure 8.1, the spinal cord derives its blood supply from a single anterior spinal artery and paired posterior spinal arteries. The anterior spinal artery is formed by the fusion of two branches from the vertebral arteries, at the level of the foramen magnum, and runs in the anterior median fissure. It supplies blood to the anterior two-thirds of the spinal cord, through which the motor tracts descend. The posterior spinal arteries supply the posterior one-third of the spinal cord, through which the sensory tracts ascend. These paired posterior spinal arteries receive supply from the posterior and inferior cerebellar arteries, the vertebral arteries, and the radicular arteries.

During its course, the anterior spinal artery receives supplemental flow, much like tributaries to a river, from upper cervical, thoracic (also known as " intercostal"), lumbar, and sacral segmental arteries (Figure 8.2). These segmental arteries are believed to be critical in the relative watershed area of the thoracolumbar spinal cord. Historically, the most important of these was thought to be the arteria radicularis magna ("artery of Adamkiewicz"), which originates between T9 and T12 in approximately 75% of individuals. Early surgical techniques emphasized the importance of preserving the artery of Adamkiewicz and other large segmental thoracic and lumbar arteries to prevent paraplegia. Even with preoperative efforts to identify the artery of Adamkiewicz and painstaking intraoperative reimplantation of this and other segmental vessels, a significant paraplegia rate occurred. Thus, recent literature has questioned the significance of the artery of Adamkiewicz and its role in the occurrence of SCI. Led by aortic surgeon Randall Griepp, one investigative group has suggested a "collateral network concept"[8] of spinal cord blood supply. This theory

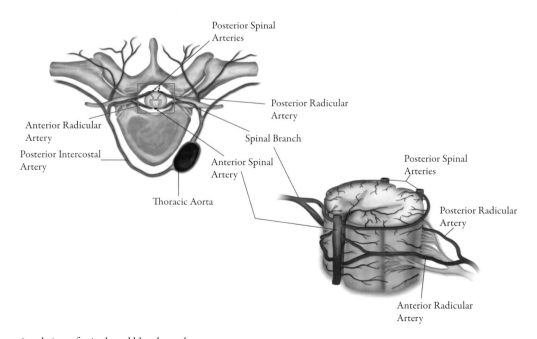

Figure 8.1 Cross-sectional view of spinal cord blood supply.

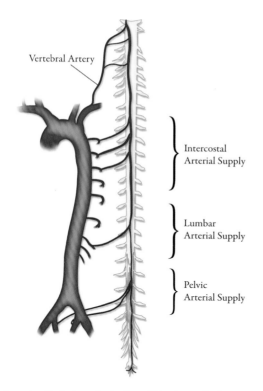

Vertebral Artery

Intercostal
Arterial Supply

Lumbar
Arterial Supply

Pelvic
Arterial Supply

Figure 8.2 Longitudinal view of spinal cord blood supply demonstrating segmental arteries.

proposes that there exists an axial network of small arteries in the spinal canal, in the perivertebral tissues, and in the paraspinous muscles that anastomose with one another and with nutrient arteries of the spinal cord. The collateral network receives input from segmental vessels, from subclavian arteries, and from branches of the hypogastric arteries. Blood supply within this network is dynamic with the ability to increase or decrease flow depending on variable factors. Compensatory changes to the network in the perioperative period may allow a patient to tolerate sacrifice of segmental arteries feeding the blood supply to the anterior spinal cord. To date, the collateral network concept has been corroborated experimentally by elegant cast studies of the spinal cord microcirculation in the pig model, which was chosen because pigs have a similar spinal cord circulation anatomy and physiology to that of humans.

Impaired blood supply to the anterior spinal artery causes the SCI associated with TA/TAA surgery. Termed "anterior spinal artery syndrome," it is, in its most severe form, marked by a flaccid paralysis, diminished sensation to hot and cold and to pin prick, but preserved fine touch and proprioception because nerve transmission through tracts residing in the posterior columns of the cord are spared. The deficit involves the lower extremities, often extending proximally to include muscles of the lower trunk. The degree of

injury can range from full paraplegia to milder paraparesis and may be asymmetric, involving one leg to a greater extent than the other. Pain symptoms may be associated as well as impaired function of bowel or bladder. Milder forms (i.e., paraparesis) may be associated with good functional recovery if treated with aggressive rehabilitation.

The surgical literature categorizes the neurologic insult according to time of onset: immediate, defined as identified upon emergence from anesthesia, or delayed, defined as occurring in the postoperative period after a period of normal lower extremity neurologic exam. The delayed form most commonly occurs early postoperatively, usually within the first 2 postoperative days,[9,10] but onset can be seen even weeks following surgery, particularly in conditions associated with hypotension. Griepp's large series of TA/TAA patients, spanning more than a decade of surgery, provides evidence that an increasing proportion of these spinal cord injuries occur in a delayed fashion and are potentially preventable with improved postoperative management.[8]

Blood supply to the spinal cord may be interrupted during surgical dissection, during aortic cross-clamp, through failure to reimplant or deliberate sacrifice of important arteries, or via occlusion of arteries by atherosclerotic emboli or endograft stent placement. Any of these mechanisms may result in cord ischemia or infarction. Secondary injury may arise from removal of the aortic cross-clamp, causing hyperemia and swelling of the spinal cord, with further compromised cord blood supply. Thrombosis, due to inflammation, hypotension, or hypoperfusion, is also a proposed mechanism of impaired perfusion to the spinal cord. These latter mechanisms may explain the phenomena of delayed neurologic deficits.

RISK FACTORS

The anatomy of spinal cord perfusion, as previously described, plays an important role in determing a patient's risk for SCI. Cord perfusion is a complex, dynamic process dependent on both collateral circulation and single segmental arteries. Temporary or permanent disruption of blood supply predisposes the spinal cord to ischemia or infarction.

Established risk factors for SCI include the location and extent of aneurysm. Highest risk occurs during repair of TAAs, which are most commonly described according to the Crawford classification (Figure 8.3). Type I describes aneurysm beginning just distal to the the left subclavian artery and ending above the renal arteries. Type II has the same beginning point but extends below the diaphragm, ending

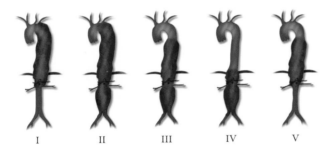

Figure 8.3 Crawford classification of thoracoabdominal aortic aneurysm with Safi's modification.

below the renal arteries. Type III describes aneurysm beginning in the descending thoracic aorta at approximately the sixth intercostal space and ending below the renal arteries. Type IV describes aneurysm below the diaphragm, beginning at the twelfth intercostal space and ending below the renal arteries. In 1995, Safi modified the classic Crawford classification, adding a fifth type, which begins at the sixth intercostal space, ends immediately above the renal arteries, and, in contemporary studies, is associated with a low risk of SCI.[11] The relationship between SCI risk and Crawford aneurysm type was demonstrated by Svensson et al.[12] in a historic series of 1,509 patients. Those patients with greatest extent TAA, Type II, had the highest incidence of SCI, 31%; incidence was 15% in Type I, 7% in Type III, and only 4% in Type IV aneurysms. Indeed, even infrarenal abdominal aortic aneurysm (AAA) repair can be complicated by SCI, occurring in an estimated 0.25% of patients.[13]

Early surgical practice for TA/TAA repair is known as "clamp-and-sew technique." As the term implies, a clamp is placed on the descending thoracic aorta while the surgeon sews vascular anastomoses as rapidly as possible because no adjunct perfusion is provided to organs or tissues that are normally fed from blood vessels distal to the clamp. Crawford's pioneering work initially recognized the association between aortic cross-clamp time and SCI; his 1993 publication[12] with colleague Svensson documented a 50% SCI rate with cross-clamp time >45 minutes. This finding led contemporary surgeons to derive operative techniques (described below) that provide perfusion to the critical segmental arteries during the period of aortic cross-clamp, thereby prolonging the tolerable ischemic time and making clamp time less important to SCI risk in the modern era.

Emergent operation and aortic rupture are consistently identified risk factors for SCI following open TA/TAA repair. Intraoperative hypotension due to blood loss with resultant diminished cord perfusion is a plausible explanation. Other factors associated with SCI include acute aortic

dissection, intraoperative hypotension, intraoperative transfusion requirement, and perioperative renal dysfunction. The extent and number of sacrificed segmental arteries during open repair is variably associated with incidence of SCI, with some investigators finding a positive correlation but others demonstrating none. Interestingly, the surgical group led by Acher had practiced a strategy of deliberate ligation of the intercostal segmental arteries, theorizing that reimplantation may cause shunt away from the spinal cord and that other factors, including collateral flow, cerebrospinal fluid pressure, and the perioperative metabolic mileu are more important to SCI risk reduction.[14] With these multiple adjuncts and deliberate intercostal ligation, the group had a low paralysis rate of 4.8%, which is comparable to the opposite technique practiced by others of segmental artery reimplantation. Nonetheless, in an effort to further reduce SCI, Acher's group incorporated selective intercostal artery reimplantation based on preoperative MR angiography and surgical inspection for patent vessels. This change in surgical practice from 2005–2008 reduced the SCI rate to 0.88%.[14]

Surgical advancement to endovascular repair of TA/TAA (TEVAR) has been shown to have a lower risk of SCI than that with open surgery. This may be attributable to greater hemodynamic stability during the procedure, less surgical insult and fewer fluid shifts, and avoidance of aortic cross-clamp. Nonetheless, in some sense the improved SCI outcomes associated with TEVAR defy anatomic explanation, because the TEVAR procedure includes stent graft coverage and occlusion of the critical segmental arteries providing spinal cord blood supply without opportunity to reimplant these vessels, as may occur during open surgical repair. The apparent nonsequitur of a lower SCI rate following TEVAR underscores the multifactorial nature of SCI, which resists simplistic etiologic explanation.

Specific to TEVAR, a risk factor for SCI includes prior aortic surgery, particularly that involving areas which might have contributed collateral flow. For example, infrarenal AAA repair may increase the risk of SCI from subsequent TEVAR due to sacrifice of important lumbar segmental vessels that, if present, might have provided collaterals to the anterior spinal artery when intercostal segmental arteries are obstructed by the thoracic stent graft. Similarly, the literature points to a higher risk of SCI in patients with obstructed internal iliac arteries as these provide important collaterals (iliolumbar and lateral sacral arteries) to the caudal segments of the spinal cord. Collateral contribution from the cervical cord blood supply may be compromised if the TEVAR procedure requires coverage of the left subclavian artery, thereby interrupting antegrade blood flow to the ipsilateral vertebral and internal thoracic artery. The length of the thoracic stent graft has also been shown to be predictive of SCI, with an increased risk seen at stent lengths >20 cm. Similar to open aortic surgery, stents that cover the distal descending thoracic aorta, interrupting blood supply to the "watershed" area (where the artery of Adamkiewicz typically arises when present), are believed to pose greater risk for SCI.

In the postoperative period, even transient periods of hypotension may result in SCI. The vascular supply to the spinal cord is particularly tenuous, vulnerable to ischemic insult, and dependent on collateral flow. Conditions that produce hypotension, including administration of antihypertensive, sedative or analgesic medications, hypovolemia, infection, or renal replacement therapy, can all result in sudden-onset SCI with devastating effects.

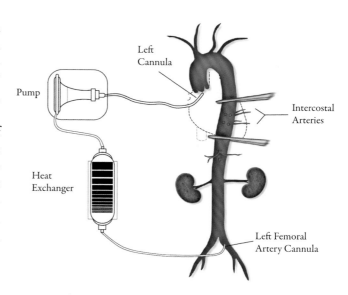

Figure 8.4 Left atrial-femoral bypass circuit, showing isolation of intercostal segmental arteries from circulation ACKNOWLEDGMENT: the authors are grateful to Samuel Rodriguez, M.D., for his artistry in Figures 8.1 to 8.4.

PREVENTIVE STRATEGIES AND TREATMENT

SURGICAL TECHNIQUES

Open surgery of the thoracic and thoracoabdominal aorta has witnessed evolution from the simple clamp-and-sew technique to current sophisticated adjuncts using either cardiopulmonary bypass (CPB) or partial heart bypass, also known as left atrial-femoral bypass (LAFB). Newer operative techniques also include 1) thoracic endovascular stents (TEVAR) and 2) "hybrid" surgery, which includes an open vascular bypass procedure combined with some form of stent graft repair. Much of this operative evolution has aimed to reduce the dreaded complication of SCI following aortic surgery. Initial preventive strategies sought to keep aortic cross-clamp time to a minimum, coupled with a competing desire to reimplant as many segmental arteries as possible. From this arose the concept of incorporating distal aortic perfusion (DAP) with retrograde flow, initially with passive (Gott) shunts to the distal aorta and more recently with left atrial-femoral bypass (LAFB). (Figure 8.4).

LAFB employs two intravascular cannulae, one inserted into the left atrium and through which oxygenated blood exits the body and flows through an extracorporeal circuit and pump, and one inserted distally into the femoral artery and through which the blood returns to the body, flowing backward into the aorta. This provides blood supply to the spinal cord in a retrograde fashion while proximal anastomoses are performed. The goal distal perfusion pressure with LAFB is 60–70 mmHg, as measured most commonly via a femoral arterial catheter or other catheter placed into the distal abdominal aorta. The technique minimizes ischemic time to the spinal cord and other vital organs (e.g., liver, kidneys) and has been shown to reduce the risk of

SCI compared to historical approaches to operative repair. Estrera et al. showed a reduction of SCI from 6.5% to 1.3% using a technique including LAFB.[15] Similarly, Conrad et al. demonstrated a significantly reduced combined risk of death and paraplegia of 2% with use of LAFB technique as compared to 9% in the clamp-and-sew cohort.[16]

HYPOTHERMIA

Hypothermia is another adjunct used to reduce the risk of SCI. Animal data suggest that metabolic rate of neurologic tissue may be reduced by approximately 6–7% for each degree Celsius reduction in temperature. Thus, reducing patient or cord temperature from 37 to 32° Celsius during surgery will, in theory, diminish metabolic rate by up to 35%. This may be achieved by allowing passive patient cooling or actively cooling via the heat exchanger (Figure 8.4) when LAFB is employed. Full CPB, with or without deep hypothermic arrest (DHA), may be the surgical approach for some patients, and is accompanied by more profound reductions in temperature (10–18° Celsius), which may protect the spinal cord. Many surgeons, however, avoid CPB and DHA unless deemed necessary by the aortic anatomy given the higher risk of other complications, including bleeding and stroke.

NEUROLOGIC MONITORING

Use of neurophysiologic monitoring such as motor evoked potentials (MEPs) and somatosensory evoked potentials

(SSEPs) has been used intra- and postoperatively to reduce risk for SCI. Given the predominant involvement of the anterior spinal cord in the pattern of injury, MEPs, although technically more challenging to perform, are more sensitive than SSEPs and are the preferred monitoring modality. The technique gained widespread adoption after Jacobs et al. published their experience with 52 high-risk patients (Crawford Type I and II aneurysm), none of whom suffered paraplegia and only one of whom had minor paraparesis, for an unprecedented paraplegia and paraparesis rate of 0 and 2%, respectively.[17] Jacobs' approach to SCI risk reduction in open TA/TAA repair employs a multimodal strategy of cerebrospinal fluid (CSF) drainage, MEP monitoring, distal aortic perfusion to >60 mmHg with LAFB, routine revascularization of intercostal and lumbar arteries between T6 and L3, and adjustment of surgical plan based on MEP response. Intraoperatively, sequential aortic clamping is practiced such that segmental arteries are excluded from perfusion while MEPs are closely monitored. If MEP amplitude diminishes by >75% from baseline during the period of exclusion, this can indicate physiologically important segmental arteries that must be rapidly reimplanted to avoid SCI. Restoration to baseline MEP amplitude following reimplantation is a reassuring sign of success. MEPs are used additionally to guide the distal aortic perfusion pressure and to set a safe blood pressure target for postoperative care. Many large-volume aortic surgical centers have subsequently published similarly favorable results with respect to SCI by incorporating a same or similar approach to Jacobs'.

PHARMACOLOGIC AGENTS

Various drugs have been suggested to have a protective effect on the spinal cord. Steroids, barbiturates, magnesium, lidocaine, and intrathecal papaverine have all been used with variable degrees of success. In the literature, the drug with the most consistently positive outcome effect is naloxone, although the predominance of literature comes from a single research group, that of Acher. For years, these investigators have employed a multimodal strategy of CSF drainage, moderate hypothermia (32–35° Celsius), thiopental to electroencephalogram (EEG) burst suppression during cross-clamp, methylprednisolone (30 mg/kg), and naloxone infusion (1 mcg/kg/h).[18] Recently published SCI rates from this group's technique have been very low (<4.8%),[14] but no widespread practice change incorporating naloxone infusion has yet been adopted by other large-volume centers. The protective mechanism of action

of naloxone is unclear but thought to involve opiate receptor antagonism of β-endorphin, which is suspected to potentiate ischemic SCI. Alternatively, some data indicate that naloxone diminishes levels of harmful excitatory neurotransmitters in the CSF following ischemic insult to the spinal cord. Currently, no consensus opinion regarding the relative value of naloxone to prevent SCI following aortic surgery exists.

CSF DRAINAGE

Sugie et al. (1957)[22] first suggested that a relationship between CSF pressure and development of paraplegia exists during surgery involving the thoracic aorta. In the only large-scale, randomized, controlled trial of CSF drainage for TAA repair, Coselli et al. used a standardized surgical approach with LAFB and showed that patients randomized to CSF drainage had a statistically significant diminished risk of SCI compared to controls.[6] Safi et al. have suggested that CSF drainage and distal aortic perfusion (DAP) decrease the incidence of SCI, especially in high-risk patients.[19] Now, with application of TEVAR to disease of the thoracic and thoracoabdominal aorta, Coselli's favorable results with CSF drainage in open surgical procedures have been extrapolated to the endovascular population. Numerous case reports and series show similarly positive results of CSF drainage in reducing SCI from TEVAR or in rescuing postoperative patients who develop injury in delayed fashion, but to date no randomized trial has been conducted in the endovascular population, nor is it likely to occur, given widespread agreement about its efficacy.

What is the protective mechanism of action of CSF drainage during surgery of the thoracic and thoracoabdominal aorta? The answer to this question has been the subject of voluminous research in the past 50 years and is still not well understood. However, most investigators endorse that CSF drainage has beneficial effects on spinal cord perfusion pressure (SCPP). SCPP is the difference between the distal mean arterial pressure (MAP) and CSF pressure (CSFP) or central venous pressure (CVP), whichever is greater. Aortic cross-clamp results in an increase of proximal aortic pressure, CVP, and CSFP, with a consequent overall decrease of SCPP. Titrated removal of CSF via a lumbar spinal drain decreases the spinal fluid pressure, augmenting SCPP and diminishing spinal cord ischemia. This effect may be of particular importance in the setting of spinal cord edema, which might occur after aortic unclamping produces reperfusion hyperemia and/or injury.

Placement, Monitoring, and Management of CSF Drains

At our institution, CSF lumbar drains are placed immediately preoperatively in an awake patient. Patient ability to perceive paresthesia lends a protective advantage, allowing the proceduralist to adjust the needle or catheter position. Some centers, however, routinely place CSF drains following the induction of general anesthesia. Sometimes this is unavoidable in conditions of emergent surgery where the patient presents after endotracheal intubation has been performed and sedatives or hypnotics have been administered. Similarly, sometimes a CSF drain that was placed in an awake patient fails to function properly intra- or postoperatively while the patient is intubated and sedated. In these situations, the treating team must weigh the relative risk of neurologic injury due to drain replacement against the possible benefits of reduced risk of SCI.

Another area of controversy is the timing of CSF drain placement. Some centers advocate preoperative placement the night before elective surgery, to allow maximal time between needle placement in the neuraxial space and intraoperative adminstration of heparin anticoagulation. Others, including our center, subscribe to a practice of drain placement in the immediate preoperative period,

with the knowledge that anesthetic preparation for procedure and surgical dissection inevitably results in an interval of several hours before heparin administration. What to do when one encounters a "bloody tap" during attempted drain placement—postpone surgery or change puncture site and approach and proceed—is an unresolved clinical problem.

The procedure is performed with strict aseptic technique (to avoid meningitis or spinal or epidural abscess) at a level below the lower end of the spinal cord (L2/3, L3/4, or L4/5 interspace) (Figure 8.5). A specific kit containing a silastic (silicon elastomer) catheter is often used, although some proceduralists prefer a standard epidural catheter (nylon or polyurethane), which is familiar and readily available and is placed into the intrathecal space. Once successfully placed and sterilely dressed, care should be taken to firmly secure the catheter to skin in order to avoid accidental dislodgement during the operative positioning of the patient.

The catheter is connected, again using aseptic technique, to a manometer or pressure transducer and simultaneously to a measuring chamber with attached collecting bag via a stopcock (Figure 8.6). Using this setup, the CSF drain may passively drain or the CSFP may be transduced and measured as determined necessary by the anesthesiologist. The zeroing point of the CSF drain transducer has generated

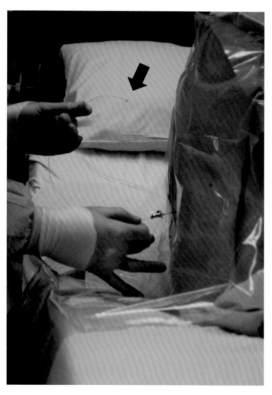

Figure 8.5 CSF drain placement. Note CSF dripping from catheter end (arrow).

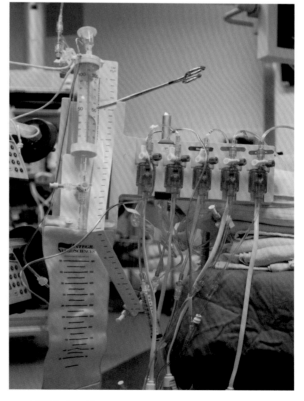

Figure 8.6 CSF drain collection apparatus.

discussion. Unlike measurement of intracranial pressure and cerebral perfusion pressure, which uses the tragus of the ear as the zero reference, lumbar CSF drains are most appropriately referenced to the phlebostatic axis in the operating room, which results in a lower measurement of spinal cord perfusion pressure and a higher measurement of CSFP than that at the tragus. Postoperatively, when the patient is likely to be nursed in a head-elevated position, we alter the zero reference to the insertion point of the drain in the lumbar spine, which we believe more accurately reflects the CSFP at the "at-risk" area of the spinal cord. This altered positioning results in greater CSF drainage than would occur if the reference point continued to be the phlebostatic axis. There is no consensus opinion, however, about the proper zero position (phlebostatic axis versus drain insertion site) for the CSF drain; practice varies by institution.[20]

CSF can be drained into the collection bag manually at fixed intervals or passively via a pop-off system in which the drainage bag is set to a certain height (usually measured in cm H_2O); the passive drainage approach automatically results in fluid drainage when the pressure exceeds a predetermined limit, in the range of 10–15 mmHg. Some institutions have protocols limiting the amount of CSF drainage to less than 10–20 ml/h, to avoid intracranial hypotension with consequent risks of intracranial hemorrhage (see below). Of note, normal CSF production is 0.2–0.7 ml/min, with total 24-hour production being 400–600 ml.

In the ICU postoperatively, CSF drainage continues to a similar CSF target pressure, with some institutions continuing to limit the volume drained as above. Should postoperative SCI manifest, dual therapy consisting of increased CSF drainage (often in 20 ml aliquots) and induced hypertension is pursued, often with immediate and sustained reversal of the paralysis or paraplegia. The duration of CSF drainage required is unclear but generally ranges from 48 to 72 hours in uncomplicated procedures. This is often extended in patients who demonstrate SCI. Precise decisions about duration of CSF drainage may be individualized to the patient, based on expected cord risk due to etiology of aortic pathology (e.g., greater with acute dissection), aneurysm anatomy and intraoperative findings (e.g., MEPs), and surgical approach (e.g., open versus endovascular). In our and many institutions, the drain is capped for 12–24 hours and the lower extremity exam closely monitored before drain removal. Careful neurologic monitoring should be continued, even after removal of the spinal drain. In the event of a delayed SCI, numerous case reports and cases series support reinstituting CSF drainage coupled with treatments to raise the blood pressure. Cheung et al.[21] describe their institutional protocol approach to managing

SCI following TEVAR as consisting of first raising MAP to 85–100 mmHg using phenylephrine or norepinephrine and, in patients who had indwelling CSF drainage, draining CSF to <10 mmHg. In patients without a functional CSF drain, if induced hypertension is ineffective at reversing the deficit, a lumbar spinal drain is replaced.

Complications of Spinal Drain

The decision to insert a spinal drain should be made deliberatively and collaboratively, involving input of both surgeon and anesthesiologist, given the potential associated risks. In elective circumstances, the procedure should be explained to the patient, including the rationale of protection from paralysis, but acknowledging the rare risk of neurologic damage attributable to the procedure itself. A review by Estrera et al. looked at 1,353 cases over 15 years of CSF drain placement for TAA surgery and reported a 99.8% technical succcess rate with a 1.5% drain-related complication rate.[22] Potential risks include infection (meningitis or spinal or epidural abscess), damage to the spinal cord or nerve roots, neuraxial hematoma, intracranial hemorrhage (ICH), retained catheter or catheter fragment upon removal, and postdural puncture headache.

Since recognition of CSF drainage benefits and general implementation, more reports of ICH complications have been seen. In a retrospective analysis of 486 lumbar drains, Wynn et al. had incidences of 1% symptomatic and 2.9% asymptomatic ICH when head CT was performed to investigate bloody CSF drainage or new-onset neurologic deficits.[23] ICH caused by CSF drainage is explained by intracranial hypotension leading to caudal displacement of the brain in the skull, including possible cerebellar tonsillar sagging and herniation, and traction on intracranial venous vessels, which may tear. The hemorrhage may manifest as subdural, subarachnoid, or intraparenchymal hemorrhage and is associated with high mortality. The identification of ICH may be heralded by blood in the CSF drainage, prompting some to recommend immediate brain imaging when this occurs. If ICH is identified, CSF drainage should be ceased by raising the drain height to a higher level (>15 mmHg) or by capping the drain until the degree of brain injury can be evaluated, weighing the risks of this complication against that of SCI. While ICH is a particularly serious complication of CSF drainage, suspected conditions that heighten this risk, including the rate and/or volume of CSF drainage, the CSFP goal, the existence of underlying cerebral atrophy or pathology, and the presence of coagulopathy, are not well defined by evidence. Admittedly, the true incidence of ICH due to CSF drainage is unknown and perhaps underreported, but it is likely less than the risk of SCI due to aortic surgery even with current good protective adjuncts.

Finally, CSF drains should not be inserted for elective surgery if there is evidence of coagulopathy or recent administration of systemic anticoagulants because of the risk of neuraxial hematoma, which may cause SCI. Similar precautions should be taken prior to removal of the catheter. In the case of emergent operation and coagulopathy, judgment regarding the relative risk–benefit profile of the procedure should guide decision making.

POSTOPERATIVE CARE

In the immediate postoperative period, the importance of avoiding hypotension cannot be overemphasized. Clear guidelines must be issued for the ICU to maintain MAP above a certain threshold, either empirically (e.g., MAP >75–85 mmHg) or as guided by thresholds established by intraoperative MEP monitoring. The exact safe blood pressure postoperatively is unknown, but it may be higher in patients with pre-existing hypertension and altered arteriolar autoregulation. Episodes of hypotension must be immediately treated with fluids, vasopressors, and correction of the inducing insult. As noted above, when a new SCI is recognized, immediate institution of induced hypertension should occur combined with CSF drainage, or, in the absence of a drainage catheter, as soon as is feasible if blood pressure augmentation alone fails to correct the deficit.

Other postoperative conditions that have been less clearly associated with the onset of delayed SCI include hypoxemia (e.g., due to pneumonia or sepsis) or, perhaps, anemia, although the specific target for perioperative hemoglobin is undetermined.

CURRENT GUIDELINES AND RECOMMENDATIONS

In 2010, a multidisciplinary task force representing the American College of Cardiology, American Heart Association, American Association for Thoracic Surgery, Society of Cardiovascular Anesthesiologists, American Stroke Association, and others published guidelines addressing the perioperative management of TA/TAA.[24] These guidelines specifically address the topic of spinal cord protection. The only therapy receiving the highest level of endorsement (Class I, meaning "should be performed") with a rating of "Level B" evidence was CSF drainage. Therapies meeting a Class IIa recommendation, meaning "reasonable

to perform," include DAP and moderate systemic hypothermia, which had Level B supportive evidence. When planning DAP, the guidelines emphasize the importance of institutional experience in selecting a technique. Adjuncts such as glucocorticoids, mannitol, intrathecal papaverine, metabolic suppression using anesthetics, and SSEPs and MEPs received a Class IIb recommendation, meaning "may be considered" on the basis of Level B evidence.

The Society for Vascular Surgery has not issued comprehensive practice guidelines addressing thoracic aortic surgery. However, in 2009, guidelines were issued regarding management of the left subclavian artery (LSA) for TEVAR.[25] For elective surgical patients, in anatomy where stent grafting requires coverage of the LSA, preoperative revascularization is *suggested*, in part to diminish the risk of SCI. Revascularization is *strongly recommended* for patients whose anatomy "compromises perfusion to critical organs." The authors acknowledge the low quality of evidence supporting both of these recommendations.

Finally, the practice advisory from the American Society of Regional Anesthesia[26] addressing neuroaxial anesthesia in the anticoagulated patient is used at our institution to guide decision making about the safety of CSF drain placement or removal in the setting of coagulopathy or anticoagulants. We apply the recommendations to the CSF drainage procedure, although the intended aim of the advisory was to address concerns for neuraxial anesthesia.

CONCLUSION

With improvements in perioperative management and in surgical techniques, the risk of SCI occurring with TAA repair has diminished considerably. Nonetheless, the potential for SCI occurring during surgery for lesions of the thoracic and thoracoabdominal aorta persists. This chapter has discussed and distilled the current evidence-based approaches to decrease SCI risk. Endovascular treatments have significantly reduced the incidence of perioperative paraplegia and paraparesis but have not eliminated risk. The future holds promise for further gains in a reduced complication rate as technological advances allow applicability of TEVAR to expanded patient populations who today can only be offered open surgery to repair aortic disease. These advances are likely to include novel fenestrated and branched-sidearm stents which may be custom fit to individual anatomic arrangement of the segmental arteries. These developments hold promise for safer treatment options in an increasingly aging population in whom thoracic aortic disease is expected to be ever more prevalent.

CONFLICT OF INTEREST STATEMENT

R.S. and R.A. have no conflicts of interest to disclose.

REFERENCES

1. Olsson C, Thelin S, Stahle E, Ekborn A, Granath F. Thoracic aortic aneurysm and dissection: increasing prevalence and improved outcomes reported in a nationwide population-based study of more than 14,000 cases from 1987 to 2002. *Circulation.* 2006;114:2611–2618.
2. Conrad MF, Cambria RP. Contemporary management of descending thoracic and thoracoabdominal aortic aneurysms: endovascular versus open. *Circulation.* 2008;117:841–852.
3. Acher C, Wynn M. Outcomes in open repair of the thoracic and thoracoabdominal aorta. *J Vasc Surg.* 2010;52(4 Suppl):3S–9S.
4. Keith CJ, Passman MA, Carignan MJ, et al. Protocol implementation of selective postoperative lumbar spinal drainage after thoracic aortic endograft. *J Vasc Surg.* 2012;55:1–9.
5. Cheung AT, Ponchettino A, McGarvey ML, et al. Strategies to manage paraplegia risk after endovascular stent repair of descending thoracic aortic aneurysms. *Ann Thorac Surg.* 2005;80:1280–1289.
6. Coselli JS, Lemaire SA, Köksoy C, Schmittling ZC, Curling PE. Cerebrospinal fluid drainge reduces paraplegia after thoracoabdominal aortic aneurysm repair: results of a randomized clinical trial. *J Vasc Surg.* 2002;35(4):631–639.
7. Conrad, MF, Ye JY, Chung TK, Davison JK, Cambria RP. Spinal cord complications after thoracic aortic surgery: long-term survival and functional status varies with deficit severity. *J Vasc Surg.* 2008;48:47–53.
8. Etz CD, Kari FA, Mueller CS, et al. The collateral network concept: a reassessment of the anatomy of spinal cord perfusion. *J Thorac Cardiovasc Surg.* 2011;141:1020–1028.
9. Ullery BW, Cheung AT, Fairman RM, et al. Risk factors, outcomes, and clinical manifestations of spinal cord ischemia following thoracic endovascular aortic repair. *J Vasc Surg.* 2011;54:677–684.
10. Estrera AL, Miller CC, Huynh TT, et al. Preoperative and operative predictors of delayed neurologic deficit following repair of thoracoabdominal aortic aneurysm. *J Thorac Cardiovasc Surg.* 2003;126:1288–1295.
11. Safi HJ, Estrera AL, Miller CC, et al. Evolution of risk for neurologic deficit after descending and thoracoabdominal aortic repair. *Ann Thorac Surg.* 2005;80:2173–2179.
12. Svensson LG, Crawford ES, Hess KR, Coselli JS, Safi HJ. Experience with 1509 patients undergoing thoracoabdominal aortic operations. *J Vasc Surg.* 1993;17:357–370.
13. Rosenthal, D. Spinal cord ischemia after abdominal aortic operation: is it preventable? *J Vasc Surg.* 1999;30:391–399.
14. Acher CW, Wynn MM, Mell MW, Tefera G, Hoch JR. A quantitative assessment of the impact of intercostal artery reimplantation on paralysis risk in thoracoabdominal aortic aneurysm repair. *Ann Surg.* 2008;248:529–540.
15. Estrera AL, Miller CC, Chen EP, et al. Descending thoracic aortic aneurysm repair: 12-year experience using distal aortic perfusion and cerebrospinal fluid drainage. *Ann Thorac Surg.* 2005;80:1290–1296.
16. Conrad MF, Ergul EA, Patel VI, et al. Evolution of operative strategies in open thoracoabdominal aneurysm repair. *J Vasc Surg.* 2011;53:1195–1201.
17. Jacobs MJ, Meylaerts SA, Haan P, et al. Strategies to prevent neurologic deficit based on motor-evoked potentials in type I and II thoracoabdominal aortic aneurysm repair. *J Vasc Surg.* 1999;29:48–59.
18. Acher CW, Wynn MM, Hoch JR, Popic P, Archibald J, Turnipseed. Combined use of cerebral spinal fluid drainage and naloxone reduces the risk of paraplegia in thoracoabdominal aneurysm repair. *J Vasc Surg.* 1994;19:236–248.
19. Safi HJ, Miller CC, Huynh TT, et al. Distal aortic perfusion and cerebrospinal fluid drainage for thoracoabdominal and descending thoracic aortic repair. *Ann Surg.* 2003;238:372–381.
20. Fedorow CA, Moon MC, Mutch WA, Grocott HP. Lumbar cerebrospinal fluid drainage for thoracoabdominal aortic surgery: rationale and practical considerations for management. *Anesth Analg.* 2010;111:46–58.
21. Cheung AT, Pochettino A, McGarvey ML, et al. Strategies to manage paraplegia risk after endovascular stent repair of descending thoracic aortic aneurysms. *Ann Thorac Surg.* 2005;80:1280–1289.
22. Estrera AL, Sheinbaum R, Miller CC, et al. Cerebrospinal fluid drainage during thoracic aortic repair: safety and current management. *Ann Thorac Surg.* 2009;88:9–15.
23. Wynn MM, Mell MW, Tefera G, Hoch JR, Acher CW. Complications of spinal fluid drainage in thoracoabdominal aortic aneurysm repair: a report of 486 patients treated from 1987 to 2008. *J Vasc Surg.* 2009;49:29–35.
24. Hiratzka LF, Bakris GL, Beckman JA, et al. 2010 ACCF/AHA/AATS/ACR/ASA/SCA/SCAI/SIR/STS/SVM guidelines for the diagnosis and management of patients with thoracic aortic disease: a report of the American College of Cardiology Foundation/American Heart Association Task Force on Practice Guidelines, American Association for Thoracic Surgery, American College of Radiology, American Stroke Association, Society of Cardiovascular Anesthesiologists, Society for Cardiovascular Angiography and Interventions, Society of Interventional Radiology, Society of Thoracic Surgeons, and Society for Vascular Medicine. *Circulation.* 2010;121:e266–e369.
25. Matsumura JS, Lee WA, Mitchell RS et al. The Society for Vascular Surgery practice guidelines: management of the left subclavian artery with thoracic endovascular aortic repair. *J Vasc Surg.* 2009;50:1155–1158.
26. Horlocker TT, Wedel DJ, Rowlingson JC, et al. Regional anesthesia in the patient receiving antithrombotic or thrombolytic therapy: American Society of Regional Anesthesia and Pain Medicine evidence-based guidelines (third edition). *Reg Anesth Pain Med.* 2010;35:64–101.

9.

NEUROPATHIC PAIN

Robert S. Griffin and Gary J. Brenner

INTRODUCTION TO THE CLINICAL PROBLEM

Anesthesiologists rarely see their patients after the second postoperative day. Surgeons typically have more prolonged duration of care for their patients, but in many cases their involvement is also limited to a relatively brief time-period surrounding the operation. This situation limits awareness of chronic postoperative pain, which typically develops over months to years following a surgical intervention. While a subjective phenomenon not often appreciated, let alone critically assessed via validated instruments, postoperative chronic pain can be disabling and may even supercede the importance of the clinical problem initially addressed by the surgical procedure.

Chronic postsurgical pain has been defined as a pain syndrome developing postoperatively with a minimum duration of 2 months.[1] An emerging concept is that chronic postoperative pain by definition must begin as an acute pain syndrome. Also, it is the underlying biology responsible for the transition from acute to chronic pain—rather than return to a resting state—that must occur and is of greatest interest. It is hoped that understanding the differences between physiological (no development of chronic pain) and pathologic responses to operation-related injury will direct development of novel therapeutic strategies.

Several separate clinical entities fall under the rubric of chronic postsurgical pain. Complex regional pain syndrome occurring after a surgical procedure may be considered a form of chronic postsurgical pain. In addition, several surgical procedures or types of injury that are repeat offenders in terms of generating postsurgical chronic pain have led to specifically named chronic postsurgical pain syndromes. Among these are postmastectomy pain syndrome, post-thoracotomy pain syndrome, posthernia repair pain syndrome, posthysterectomy pain syndrome, postlaminotomy syndrome, and phantom limb pain. So-called failed back surgery syndrome does not neatly fall within the chronic postsurgical pain definition because it encompasses a large group of procedures performed with the intention of alleviating an underlying pain problem.

Currently, the literature on chronic postsurgical pain consists predominantly of epidemiologic studies of incidence, prevalence, outcomes, and risk factors for chronic postsurgical pain within the context of specific surgical procedures. As a result, much is known about the problem from a phenomenological standpoint. There is an extensive parallel literature regarding the mechanisms of pain—really nociceptive sensitization—related to nerve injury and inflammation in preclinical models, primarily rodents. Many of these mechanisms, such as peripheral and central sensitization, are surmised to underlie the development of chronic postsurgical pain in humans. Whether this assumption is correct remains unknown. One particular distinction between the preclinical literature and the phenomenon as it occurs in the clinical setting is the observation that most rodent studies concern a discrete lesion that either produces a potent inflammatory response or a single definable injury of a major nerve that produces a dramatic and high-prevalence pain response often spanning the remaining lifespan of the animal, which in the experimental setting typically encompasses a few days or weeks. In contrast, human postoperative pain occurs sporadically, develops after surgical technique optimized to minimize or avoid tissue injury, and persists over a widely varying time frame of a few months to a few years to decades. In addition, it is not at all obvious that the nociceptive hypersensitivity displayed by rodents is similar to the pain experience described by human patients.

With that disclaimer in mind, we will review several of the processes that may be important for the induction and maintenance of persistent pain states. Pain may fall into several categories. *Nociceptive pain* may be considered "ordinary" or nonsensitized nonpathologic pain that results from the response of the peripheral somatosensory system to a high-threshold stimulus. *Inflammatory pain* refers to a state of heightened pain sensitivity that results from the alteration of the stimulus–response properties of the peripheral and central nervous system in the setting of an inflammatory state. Inflammatory pain may be brief or protracted, primarily related to the duration of the underlying inflammatory state. *Neuropathic pain* consists of pain related to peripheral nerve injury, and includes both spontaneous pain and heightened sensitivity to peripheral stimuli. *Central pain* includes pain that results from central nervous system injury. Pathologic pain states, including neuropathic, central, and inflammatory pain, are characterized by *allodynia*, in which ordinarily nonpainful stimuli are perceived as painful; *hyperalgesia*, in which already painful stimuli feel more painful; and *spontaneous pain*, in which pain is experienced in the absence of a peripheral stimulus. *Chronic pain* describes the persistent subjective pain experience of a patient, which may or may not depend on an ongoing response to a nociceptive stimulus. A persistent pain state depends on the persistence of the painful stimulus, the transmission of information about the nociceptive stimulus to the central nervous system, plasticity of the peripheral and central nervous system transmission and processing systems, and the patient's psychological state. In some cases, a pain state may be stimulus independent as a result of plastic changes in the nervous system resulting in spontaneous or ectopic neuronal excitability. An enhanced state of excitability may result from altered signal transduction in the periphery due to inflammatory cell–cell signaling that alters nociceptive sensory thresholds, or from the massive array of anatomic and physiological modifications in the sensory system evoked by nerve injury. Most of the typical chronic postsurgical pain conditions are thought to

rely primarily on the somatic sensory system; however, there certainly must be alterations in visceral pain sensitivity (e.g., chronic abdominal pain following an operation) that contribute depending on the operative injury.

The trauma associated with even the most meticulous surgical technique will result in localized inflammation within the incised tissue. This inflammatory process along with surgical nerve injury (either macroscopic or microscopic) may potentially contribute to chronic postsurgical pain. A number of signaling systems may initiate the inflammatory response that follows surgical tissue trauma. The signaling mediators associated with blood clotting and platelet degranulation may be important initiators; platelets provide a source of multiple proinflammatory cytokines such as histamine, serotonin, eicosanoids, platelet-derived growth factor, and transforming growth factor-beta, several of which directly increase the nociceptive sensitivity of peripheral terminals. The fibrin constituent of a blood clot also acts as a chemoattractant for migratory neutrophils, macrophages, and fibroblasts. The complement cascade, a component of the innate immune system, likely is also activated in response to surgical incision. The C5a and C3a anaphylotoxin signaling peptides released by complement activation are important inflammatory mediators. C5a in particular has been demonstrated in preclinical studies to have an important role in peripheral nociceptive sensitization.[2] Peripheral sensitization related to alteration of peripheral terminal sensitivity in the context of an inflammatory response likely accounts for pain hypersensitivity in the acute state in the immediate vicinity of surgical trauma.

Direct injury—that is, physical trauma—to peripheral nerves undoubtedly constitutes an important stimulus for the development of chronic postsurgical pain. Primary sensory neurons, the sensory component of peripheral nerves, are pseudounipolar cells with cell bodies in the dorsal root ganglia (DRG) of the spinal cord, or in brainstem nuclei in the case of cranial nerves. These neurons extend a single axon that bifurcates to give rise to a central branch innervating the spinal cord or brain, and a peripheral branch that innervates the skin or other tissues (e.g., sclera, muscle) or the viscera. There are several separate populations of DRG neurons that may be distinguished according to axon diameter, axon myelination, and the array of transductive receptors, growth factor receptors, and ion channels that they express. These separate populations of DRG neurons will respond to specific modalities of peripheral stimulus, such as heat, chemical, or mechanical stimulation. Following peripheral nerve injury, extensive physiological changes occur in DRG neurons, thought to be induced by loss of trophic support provided by the innervated target, exposure of the injured axons to debris left by the Wallerian degeneration of the distal portion of the nerve, and rapid ion flux across the areas of membrane disrupted by injury.[3] These activating signals lead to fundamental alterations in primary sensory neuron physiology that include changes in gene expression, associated with altered patterns of neuropeptide synthesis and altered electrical activity. These alterations in DRG neuronal gene expression may persist over time and generate a persistently facilitated pain state. This is a form of "peripheral sensitization."

In addition to the increased excitability of the peripheral sensory system, the central nervous system is likely to be an important locus of altered physiology that may explain chronic postsurgical pain. This phenomenon is often referred to as "central sensitization." Central nervous system responses were long thought to have a role in "causalgia," a chronic pain state following major limb trauma now termed "complex regional pain syndrome type II." As written by S. Weir Mitchell, the American neurologist and Civil War battlefield surgeon, in 1872, "Nerve injuries may also cause pain which, owing to inexplicable reflex transfers in the centres, may be felt in remote tissues outside of the region which is tributary to the wounded nerve."[4] More recent experiments extending over the past three to four decades have demonstrated that sensitized responses of the central nervous system are a critical component of experimental postinjury pain hypersensitivity in animals.[5]

Somatosensory neurons provide afferent innervation to the dorsal horn of the spinal cord and to the brain. The dorsal horn is the site of initial synaptic transmission in the nociceptive spinothalamic tract pathway and is likely to be an important locus for the phenomenon of central sensitization. The dorsal horn of the spinal cord may be anatomically (and functionally) divided into 10 Rexed lamina (Figure 9.1). Peripheral nociceptors predominantly innervate the superficial lamina, I and II, while low-threshold mechanosensitive fibers predominantly innervate deeper lamina (Figure 9.1). Secondary nociceptive neurons residing within the superficial lamina have multiple modality-specific subtypes, whereas the deeper lamina secondary neurons are predominantly wide dynamic-range cells responsive to multiple stimulus modalities.[6] Following peripheral nerve injury, many of the physiological properties of the spinal cord dorsal horn change. For example, there is an increase in the proportion of cells in superficial lamina II—typically the target of nociceptive afferents—that show polysynaptic responses to low-threshold stimulus.[7] Effectively, the superficial dorsal horn acquires responsiveness to low-threshold (e.g., light touch) stimuli. Thus, the heightened pain responses observed in pathologic pain states, such as

allodynia, hyperalgesia, and spontaneous pain, may in part be explained by these alterations in central nervous system function. Numerous mechanisms have been investigated as potential explanation for this phenomenon, such as anatomic sprouting of low-threshold afferents, modified excitability of dorsal horn transmission neurons or inhibitory interneurons, synaptic long-term potentiation, and modulation by altered function of microglia and astrocytes.

Interestingly, peripheral nerve injury evokes extensive immunologic alterations in the peripheral nerve and in the spinal cord and perhaps even the brain.[8] Prominent microglial activation in the spinal cord occurs following peripheral nerve injury. Signal transduction in activated spinal cord microglia is likely to be important for the central sensitization that occurs after peripheral nerve injury. Intrathecal administration of several different agents that inhibit signal transduction pathways (ERK, p38 MAP kinase) activated in spinal microglia can reverse postinjury pain sensitization.[9] In addition, microglial toll-like receptor 4 seems to be necessary for tactile allodynia induced by peripheral nerve injury, microglial upregulation of activation markers, and upregulation of mRNA for multiple proinflammatory cytokines.[10] Gene expression analysis has demonstrated that upregulation of inflammatory mediators within the spinal cord dorsal horn may persist for a relatively long period of time, in the rat extending to at least 40 days postinjury. It seems that numerous mechanisms acting at the initial injury site, within the peripheral nervous system, or in the central

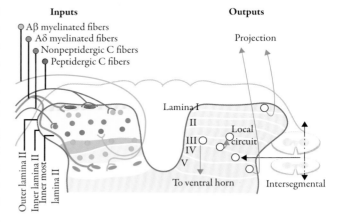

Figure 9.1 This figure demonstrates the lamina in the spinal cord dorsal horn. Small diameter C nociceptive fibers (red) as well as A delta nociceptive fibers (purple) predominantly innervate the superficial lamina of the dorsal horn, where they transmit peripheral information to ascending projection neurons (red) as well as locally communicating interneurons (green). Low threshold A beta fibers (orange) predominantly ascend directly in the dorsal column but also give rise to fibers that project to the deeper laminae of the dorsal horn FROM: Wainger, B and Brenner GJ. "Mechanisms of Chronic Pain" in Longnecker, D, Brown, DL, Newman, M, and Zapol, W. Anesthesiology, Second Edition. 2012. Mc Graw Hill Professional.

nervous system—spinal cord and brain—may account for chronic postsurgical pain syndromes.

INCIDENCE AND OUTCOMES

Chronic postsurgical pain occurs following a large variety of surgical interventions, and the duration and morbidity associated with the pain state may vary widely according to the particular surgical procedure. Even for the same procedure, the surgical approach can make a substantial difference in the likelihood of chronic postsurgical pain. For example, in a large study of chronic pain after hernia repair, at 5 years postrepair, 9.4% of patients reported chronic pain following a laparoscopic approach, while 18.8% reported pain following an open (Liechtenstein) repair.[11]

The surgical procedures listed in Table 9.1 do not represent an inclusive list. For example, chronic pain after abdominal surgery such as Roux en Y gastric bypass may represent a relatively underrecognized form of chronic postsurgical pain. In one prospective cohort study of patients 4 years postoperatively from hepatic, pancreas, biliary, or bowel surgery, 18% reported chronic pain.

There are relatively few long-term prospective studies of chronic postoperative pain. Consequently, the risk of pain-related comorbidity for a given patient undergoing an operation remains relatively unknown. Within the posthernia repair pain literature, it does appear that the incidence of chronic pain decreases over time, which is encouraging, but it remains unknown whether there is an eventual plateau or whether all of these patients recover from their chronic pain condition. In one study, patients with postmastectomy chronic pain who reported chronic postsurgical pain in 1996 also reported pain when surveyed in 2002, with mean postoperative time of 9 years; 48% of responding women with chronic postoperative pain eventually experienced resolution of pain.[12]

Table 9.1 **REPORTED INCIDENCE OF CHRONIC POSTSURGICAL PAIN**

TYPE OF PROCEDURE	INCIDENCE OF PAIN
Hernia repair	11–21% (1 year later) 9–19% (5 years later)
Mastectomy	20–50%
Hysterectomy	5–32%
Thoracotomy	25–60%
Sternotomy	11–56%

TABLE REFERENCES: Hernia repair[11,25]; mastectomy[26]; hysterectomy[27]; thoracotomy[28]; sternotomy.[29]

RISK FACTORS

Extensive studies have been performed in an attempt to identify risk factors that may help predict patients susceptible to chronic postsurgical pain so that they may either choose to avoid elective operations or obtain optimal postoperative care. There are several limitations to these studies. Prominently, most of them are retrospective, limiting strength of many of the conclusions that may be drawn.[13] In addition, many of the putative risk factors that have been identified thus far are nonintervenable, representing underlying demographic characteristics of the patient group.

Several different types of risk factor for chronic postoperative pain have been considered. Several factors that have been identified as important for chronic postsurgical pain include intensity of baseline pain, relatively young age within study population, and occurrence of postoperative complication.[14] Intensity and other properties of acute postoperative pain have also been investigated as potential risk factors for chronic postoperative pain. There is not a single answer to this question across types of surgical procedure. Psychological factors, such as level of catastrophizing, have been associated with an increased risk of chronic postoperative pain.[15] One large study of postoperative pain after breast cancer surgery demonstrated risk factors for chronic postsurgical pain including young age, adjuvant radiotherapy, and axillary as opposed to sentinel lymph node dissection.[16] Pain problems distal to the surgical site also predicted an increased likelihood of persistent pain at the surgical site.

Characteristics of the surgical procedure that affect the likelihood of developing chronic postsurgical pain, such as sentinel as opposed to axillary lymph node dissection, have been studied. These characteristics are of great importance because of those considered, surgical technique is often the only factor presently amenable to modification. Many of the other potential risk factors that have been identified thus far are essentially immutable, such as genetic background and age. Of the potentially modifiable risk factors, the chain of causality remains ambiguous in most cases: does worse acute postoperative pain cause chronic postoperative pain, or is worse acute postoperative pain a manifestation of an underlying state that also gives rise to the eventual development of chronic postoperative pain? While the same reasoning may also apply to surgical technique, given that an underlying factor may determine both the choice of the surgical procedure and the occurrence of chronic postsurgical pain (such as preprocedure disease burden), this appears relatively less likely to apply for all surgical decisions.

Recently, an increasing number of studies have begun to investigate genetic factors that may affect the development of chronic postsurgical pain. There are several avenues through which a patient's genetic background may affect postsurgical pain. Patients may differ in genetic susceptibility in baseline pain sensitivity, which is carried forward to the postoperative period. Or, patients may vary in the genetic predisposition to develop a chronic pain state. Patients may also vary genetically in terms of responsiveness to some of the commonly used medications or interventions intended to treat the painful condition. Finally, genetic variation among patients may affect the underlying disease process that the surgical procedure is intended to correct and, as such, may indirectly alter the parameters of the surgical procedure.[17]

Several genes have been identified that may affect the tendency to develop persistent pain following a surgical procedure. Using a candidate gene approach based on the results from microarray, molecular, and behavioral data from rodents, Tegeder et al. (2006)[18] identified a polymorphism in the gene for GTP cyclohydrolase I as a potential factor affecting the tendency to experience pain after surgery intended to treat low back pain. GTP cyclohydrolase catalyzes the rate-limiting step in the synthesis of tetrahydrobiopterin, a cofactor that in turn is required for catecholamine, serotonin, and nitric oxide synthesis. More recently, a similar approach has implicated polymorphisms in the gene *Kcns1* encoding a potassium channel subunit, Kv9.1, as a potential factor in some types of chronic postsurgical pain.[19] While this channel is expressed in rodent DRG neurons and prominently downregulated after peripheral nerve injury, its precise function in pain and nociception remains unknown.

In addition to genes that may affect the tendency to develop postoperative pain, there is increasing evidence that gene polymorphisms may affect the response to therapy. It has long been known that variants in the cytochrome P450 system can alter drug metabolism from patient to patient. Opioid metabolism is no exception, and these genetic variants can have an important impact on postoperative pain management. Carriers of the CYP2D6 ultra-rapid metabolizer genotype can rapidly convert codeine into morphine, resulting in what is ordinarily a weak opioid acting as a relatively potent agent.[20] More recently, studies of the gene encoding the mu opioid receptor indicate that polymorphisms in this gene may affect patients' postoperative opioid requirement.[17] The intricacy of the numerous processes that may affect pain sensitivity are highlighted by a recent study demonstrating that polymorphisms in the vasopressin 1A receptor can alter capsaicin-induced pain levels, but only in patients reporting psychological stress while undergoing the experimental challenge.[21]

PREVENTIVE STRATEGIES AND TREATMENT

Prevention of chronic postsurgical pain has primarily focused on (a) modification of the surgical procedure to reduce or limit nerve injury or tissue trauma, and (b) modification of anesthetic technique and perioperative pain management in the hopes of altering the development of nervous system plasticity that likely underlies the long-term maintenance of a chronic pain state. Optimizing acute pain management is certainly an important component of ensuring an ideal perioperative experience for the patient. Whether improved postoperative pain control reduces the tendency to develop chronic postsurgical pain or whether easier postoperative pain control identifies a subtype or mechanistically related group of patients who are intrinsically unlikely to develop chronic postsurgical pain remains unknown.

Several groups have investigated whether specific agents thought to modulate neuropathic pain may result in a prolonged reduction in postoperative acute and/or chronic pain. Extensive animal research has implicated NMDA-type glutamate receptors in nociceptive sensitization. As a result, ketamine, which antagonizes the NMDA glutamate receptor and also has analgesic properties, is an intriguing candidate for a pain-protective analgesic strategy. Although at least one study has demonstrated reduced opioid use at 6 weeks in patients randomized to receive intraoperative ketamine, this finding and its durability remain to be validated as a primary outcome in a large study.[22] Several studies have indicated that perioperative administration of either gabapentin or pregabalin is associated with decreased postsurgical pain;[23] however, the data are insufficient to support alterations in clinical practice. The investigation of specific long-term outcomes in association with particular perioperative interventions remains widely open for future investigation.

As discussed, the pathophysiology of chronic postoperative pain almost certainly includes multiple underlying mechanisms, involving highly regulated bidirectional interactions between the nervous and immune systems, that occur in both the peripheral and central nervous systems. In contrast to other general chronic pain disorders, there is relatively little to guide therapy that is specific to chronic postsurgical pain. Optimally, management of these conditions will involve a multidisciplinary approach that may include pharmacologic, interventional, and rehabilitative modalities. Numerous clinical personnel may be involved in this process and may include the patient's surgeon, pain medicine physicians, psychologists, psychiatrists, and physical therapists, among others. The importance of the longitudinal involvement of the patient's surgeon in this process cannot be overstated, both for ongoing surveillance and re-evaluation of the original surgical problem and for helping the patient avoid the sense of abandonment and loss of interest that may accrue from a chronic postsurgical pain condition.

Pharmacologic agents are widely used in the management of chronic postsurgical pain. They are typically used on the basis of management of neuropathic pain conditions in general, with relatively little information to guide specific treatment selection for particular postsurgical pain conditions. Unfortunately, there are virtually no high-quality data to guide drug treatment selection in this arena. In general terms, the useful armamentarium consists of tricyclic antidepressants, α_2-δ calcium channel subunit ligands (i.e., gabapentin and pregabalin), other antiepileptics, nonsteroidal anti-inflammatory drugs, opioids, and local anesthetics. The use of chronic opioid therapy for persistent postoperative pain remains a prominent and controversial issue among experts in the field. There are substantial potential risks of chronic opioid therapy, including altered endocrine and immune function, possible opioid-induced hyperalgesia, development of psychological dependence, and potential harm from direct opioid side effects. Because opioids are essentially the mainstay of acute postoperative pain management, commonly necessary even in patients at high risk for complications from opioid therapy due to prior history of addiction or substance misuse, physicians will inevitably encounter patients who linger on chronic opioid therapy less out of a decision-making process by any specific physician than out of the inertia of the patient's pain condition. As with neuropathic pain medications, there are no truly long-term studies of outcomes or efficacy for opioids in chronic postsurgical pain.

In addition to pharmacologic approaches, there are a variety of other modalities that may be considered for treatment of chronic postsurgical pain. Where appropriate, neuromodulation approaches such as spinal cord or peripheral nerve stimulation may be considered; the latter remains an investigational approach. Spinal cord stimulation may have utility in the management of chronic postlaminotomy pain syndrome[24]—a major form of chronic pain. In patients who are refractory to pharmacotherapy and have pain that proves nonresolving over time, close attention to a patient's mental health is essential given the substantial potential for psychiatric comorbidity.

RECOMMENDATIONS

As should be apparent from this review, understanding of the epidemiology and pathophysiology of chronic postsurgical pain syndromes is in its infancy. Thus, guidelines for prevention and management of chronic postsurgical pain are based largely on knowledge of treatment of other persistent pain conditions. We consider the following recommendations to be reasonable:

1. Include the potential for chronic postsurgical pain as part of informed consent.

2. In patients who are at high risk for chronic postsurgical pain, provide adequately long-term follow-up to ensure that acute postoperative pain resolves.

3. In patients who develop chronic postsurgical pain, consider referral to subspecialty care—for example, pain medicine, neurology—as appropriate.

CONCLUSION

Chronic postsurgical pain is a common, yet generally underappreciated consequence of a wide variety of surgical procedures. The risk factors, pathophysiology, and optimal management are all incompletely understood, with much of present understanding reliant on studies of neuropathic pain conditions. Mitigation of chronic postsurgical pain represents a major unmet medical need. Several general questions deserve further investigation. Are there cases in which the risk of chronic postsurgical pain may argue for avoiding a surgical procedure? Can chronic postsurgical pain be reduced or avoided via optimal surgical technique or perioperative anesthetic management? What are the best practices for management of patients in whom chronic postsurgical pain develops? At present there are no definitive answers to these questions.

CONFLICT OF INTEREST STATEMENT

G.J.B. and R.S.G. have no conflicts of interest to disclose.

REFERENCES

1. Macrae WA, Davies HTO. Chronic postsurgical pain. In: Crombie IK, Croft PR, Linton SJ, LeResche L, and Von Korff, M, eds. *Epidemiology of Pain*. Seattle: IASP Press; 1999:125–142.

2. Liang DY, Li X, Shi X, et al. The complement component C5a receptor mediates pain and inflammation in a postsurgical pain model. *Pain*. 2012;153(2):366–372.
3. Makwana M, Raivich G ."Molecular mechanisms in successful peripheral regeneration." *FEBS J*. 2005; 272(11): 2628–2638.
4. Mitchell, SW. *Injuries of nerves and their consequences*. New York: Dover;1872 (1965 ed).
5. Woolf CJ 1983. "Evidence for a central component of post-injury pain hypersensitivity." *Nature*. 1983; 306(5944): 686–688.
6. Craig AD 2003. "Pain mechanisms: labeled lines versus convergence in central processing." *Annu Rev Neurosci* 2003; (26): 1–30.
7. Kohno T, Moore KA, Baba H, Woolf CJ. Peripheral nerve injury alters excitatory synaptic transmission in lamina II of the rat dorsal horn. *J Physiol*. 2003;548(1):131–138.
8. Abbadie C, Bhangoo S, De Koninck Y, Malcangio M, Melik-Parsadaniantz S, White FA. Chemokines and pain mechanisms. *Brain Res Rev*. 2009;60(1):125–134.
9. Ji RR, Gereau RW 4th, Malcangio M, Strichartz GR. MAP kinase and pain. *Brain Res Rev*. 2008;60(1):135–148.
10. Tanga FY, Nutile-McMenemy N, DeLeo JA. The CNS role of Toll-like receptor 4 in innate neuroimmunity and painful neuropathy. *Proc Natl Acad Sci U S A*. 2005;102(16):5856–5861.
11. Eklund A, et al. Chronic pain 5 years after randomized comparison of laparoscopic and Lichtenstein inguinal hernia repair. *Br J Surg*. 2010;97(4):600–608.
12. Macdonald L, et al. Long-term follow-up of breast cancer survivors with post-mastectomy pain syndrome. *Br J Cancer*. 2005;92(2):225–230.
13. Kehlet H, Rathmell JP. Persistent postsurgical pain. *Anesthesiology*. 2010;112: 514–515.
14. Fränneby U, et al. Risk factors for long-term pain after hernia surgery. *Ann Surg*. 2006;244(2):212–219.
15. Khan RS, et al. Catastrophizing: a predictive factor for postoperative pain. *Am J Surg*. 2011;201(1):122–131.
16. Gärtner R, et al. Prevalence of and factors associated with persistent pain following breast cancer surgery. *JAMA*. 2009;302(18):1985–1992.
17. Allegri M, De Gregori M, Niebel T, et al. Pharmacogenetics and postoperative pain. *Minerva Anestesiol*. 2012;76(11):937–944.
18. Tegeder I, et al. GTP cyclohydrolase and tetrahydrobiopterin regulate pain sensitivity and persistence. *Nat Med*. 2006;12(11):1269–1277.
19. Costigan M, et al. Multiple chronic pain states are associated with a common amino acid-changing allele in KCNS1. *Brain*. 2010;133(9):2519–2527.
20. Lötsch J. Genetic variability of pain perception and treatment—clinical pharmacological implications. *Eur J Clin Pharmacol*. 2011;67(6):541–551.
21. Mogil JS, et al. Pain sensitivity and vasopressin analgesia are mediated by a gene-sex-environment interaction. *Nat Neurosci*. 2011;14(12):1569–1573.
22. Loftus RW, et al. Intraoperative ketamine reduces perioperative opiate requirement in opiate-dependent patients with chronic back pain undergoing back surgery. *Anesthesiology*. 2010;113(3):639–646.
23. Grosu I, de Kock M. New concepts in acute pain management: strategies to prevent chronic postsurgical pain, opioid-induced hyperalgesia, and outcome measures. *Anesthesiol Clin*. 2011;29(2):311–327.
24. North RB, Kidd DH, Farrokhi F, Piantadosi SA. Spinal cord stimulation versus repeated lumbosacral spine surgery for chronic pain: a randomized, controlled trial. *Neurosurgery*. 2005;56(1):98–106.
25. Messenger DE, Aroori S, Vipond MN. Five-year prospective follow-up of 430 laparoscopic totally extraperitoneal inguinal hernia repairs in 275 patients. *Ann R Coll Surg Engl*. 2010;92(3):201–205.
26. Vadivelu N, et al. Pain after mastectomy and breast reconstruction. *Am Surg* 2008;74(4):285–296.
27. Brandsborg B, et al. Chronic pain after hysterectomy. *Acta Anaesthesiol Scand*. 2008;52(3):327–331.
28. Wildgaard K, Ravn J, Kehlet H. Chronic post-thoracotomy pain: a critical review of pathogenic mechanisms and strategies for prevention. *Eur J Cardiothorac Surg*. 2009;36(1):170–180.
29. Mazzeffi M, Khelemsky Y. Poststernotomy pain: a clinical review. *J Cardiothorac Vasc Anesth*. 2011;25(6):1163–1178.

PART III

NERVE

10.

PERIPHERAL NERVE INJURY

Marnie B. Welch and Chad M. Brummett

INTRODUCTION TO THE CLINICAL PROBLEM

Perioperative peripheral nerve injury is a serious complication, accounting for significant patient morbidity. It represents the third most commonly recognized cause of anesthesia litigation and 16% of all American Society of Anesthesiologists (ASA) closed claims.[1] In the ASA closed-claims database, the frequency of serious events (death, brain injury) has been decreasing, but the claims for nerve injury have not decreased relative to more serious claims and thus still represent a significant percentage of the closed claims.[2]

Excluding obvious surgical causes, such as direct trauma, retraction, postoperative casting, and compressive wraps, perioperative nerve injuries can occur in a variety of ways, often being multifactorial and without a clear mechanism. Nerve injury can occur by direct trauma, either with placement of intravenous and intra-arterial lines or with peripheral nerve blocks and neuraxial techniques. Otherwise, neuropathy is generally thought to be related to positioning. The administration of anesthetics and muscle relaxants temporarily removes the patient's ability to prevent extremes of body position or excessive pressure leading to injury. Irrespective of the mechanical etiology, there are multiple pathologic mechanisms at the physiological level of the nerve that lead to patient symptoms: direct trauma, stretch, compression, generalized ischemia, metabolic abnormalities, and environmental abnormalities. For example,

most peripheral nerves are intolerant of prolonged stretch beyond 5% of normal resting length.[3] Disrupted blood flow in anesthetized patients leads to intraneural hemorrhage, ischemia, and/or necrosis, potentially resulting in elevated intraneural venous pressure and edema. Certain patients with pre-existing conditions are more susceptible to this trauma to the nervous system – whether their nerves are chronically dysfunctional or they have a general condition that compromises blood flow. Also, certain metabolic and environmental conditions, such as hypoxia and cold, can contribute to dysfunctional axonal conduction and demyelination, resulting in patient symptoms.[4]

The severity of nerve injury and long-term structural damage is dependent on a combination of the pre-existing condition of the nerve and the degree of stretch and compression. Mild injuries occur with a temporary interruption of the blood supply, such as with minor compression when the nerve is draped over a firm surface.[4] Ischemia occurs in the immediate anatomic area, leading to a conduction block. This temporary conduction block, whether motor or sensory, recovers rapidly within minutes to hours or perhaps a few days. Patients may or may not report any problem because it resolves or they are still under the sedative effects of general anesthesia, opioids, or other medications. These injuries likely account for the higher incidence of nerve injury in prospective studies, in which patients are asked directly about new neurologic symptoms after surgery.

More severe nerve injuries involve damage to the myelin and are even more serious if the axon was not preserved. As proposed by Seddon in 1942,[5] *neuropraxic* injuries are from a moderate conduction block in which the myelin sheath is damaged but the rest of the nerve is intact. These injuries mostly commonly occur with compression or stretch injuries and take approximately 4–6 weeks to recover as the myelin regenerates. Nerve fibers with little connective tissue seem more susceptible to injury. Electromyography (EMG) shows slowing or a conduction block.

In the next level of severity, *axonotmesis* occurs either by severe crush or traction, and the axon is destroyed. The recovery is slow and may be incomplete, as it is reliant on collateral reinnervation from surrounding nerves, preservation of Schwann cells to assist in regrowth, or axonal regrowth. The recovery time is 3–12 months, as a nerve grows approximately 1 mm/day. These injuries are rare but more devastating to patients. EMG shows that the amplitude of the compound action potentials is reduced or, with complete axonal loss, denervational changes exist.

The most severe injury, *neurotmesis,* occurs with total disruption of the axon and connective tissue elements; this is often related to the surgery itself. The growing axons have no guide to the correct peripheral target and there is no opportunity for regeneration. If function or partial function is to be regained, then surgery is often required. With this level of injury, EMG reveals total loss of distal segment function.

INCIDENCE AND OUTCOME

When describing neuropathy in the perioperative period, the etiologies can broadly be broken into two categories: 1) those associated with patient positioning or surgical traction in routine anesthetic care, and 2) those assumed to be procedural complications with invasive anesthesia procedures, including regional anesthesia and other invasive procedures (e.g., arterial line placement). The reported incidence of perioperative nerve injury following anesthesia is low, ranging from 0.016% to14.0% depending on patient populations, types of anesthetics, and types of nerve injury.[6–11] The range in incidence is due to multiple factors, including varying definitions of nerve injuries, sample size, and study methodology. Ulnar nerve injuries have been best studied and have an incidence of 0.04%.[9] Given that sensory neuropathies are far more common than motor injuries and generally resolve over time without intervention,[8,10–13] the reported incidence likely underestimates the true occurrence.

Although nerve injury following regional anesthesia is a concern in the anesthesia community, there have been few prospective studies. In France, using a self-report hotline for anesthesiologists, Auroy et al.[14] found very few neurologic complications after regional anesthesia. This study is often falsely labeled as prospective. Brull et al.[6] completed a meta-analysis in 2007, noting an incidence of 0.038% for spinal anesthesia, 0.022% for epidurals, 2.48% for interscalene blocks, 1.48% for axillary blocks, and 0.34% femoral blocks. The results of this meta-analysis could be skewed by the disproportionate size of the Auroy study. Three prospective studies of neurologic sequelae after interscalene brachial plexus block all reported a much higher incidence, ranging from 8% to 14%.[15–17] Injuries in obstetric practice range from 0.008% to 0.5% from all causes, not just those suspected from regional anesthesia and analgesia.[11] In the most recent review, by Capdevila et al., of 1,416 peripheral nerve catheters, the incidence of hypoesthesia or numbness was 3% and 2.2%, respectively, after 5 days; the longer-lasting ones were followed (0.2%) with subsequent resolution ranging from 36 hours to 10 days.[18] Most incidence data have been obtained from adult populations; evidence in the pediatric population is usually limited to case reports.

It is important to note that there have been no studies randomizing patients to nerve block or general anesthesia, thereby making it impossible to assess the additional risk from regional anesthesia. Some studies have tried to differentiate the symptoms likely associated with nerve blockade from other potential causes (e.g., positioning, traction) and have found that the distribution of symptoms does not often correlate with the nerves or plexus blocked.[16,17] Jacob et al.[12,13] found no association between regional anesthesia and nerve injury following total knee and hip arthroplasty. In perhaps the only data supportive of a lack of association between peripheral nerve blockade and nerve injury after total knee arthroplasty, the authors demonstrated that despite a sharp increase in regional anesthesia in recent years for total knee arthroplasty, the incidence of postoperative neurologic sequelae in this cohort has remained stable.[12]

TIMING AND QUALITY OF PERIOPERATIVE NEUROPATHIES

In studies of large patient populations, either sensory symptoms or sensorimotor symptoms appear to be more common, and motor symptoms are least common.[8,10–13] For example, in a study of 380,680 patients with perioperative peripheral nerve injury, two-thirds were sensory, 27% were combined motor and sensory, and only 16% were isolated motor injury.[10] However, injuries in the closed-claims database were more likely to include motor changes,[2,10] suggesting either a greater source of disability to the patient or worse recovery profile.

Upper extremity injury usually predominates over lower extremity injury, as it does in the closed-claims database and in large patient populations, by a ratio of 3:2.[2,10] Reported injuries exists in essentially all major peripheral nerves. Recurrent laryngeal nerve palsies can occur for a variety of reasons, including laryngeal mask airway (LMA) placement and transesophageal echocardiographic probe placement. Rare injuries have been reported, including facial nerve injury thought to be due to mask ventilation, lingual nerve injury from the endotracheal tube or LMA, pudendal nerve injury from traction, and supraorbital injury with a face harness.

The natural history of perioperative peripheral nerve injuries is unclear because of the varying degree of follow-up. In a meta-analysis of injuries after regional anesthesia, the rate of permanent injury was 0–4.2:10,000 after central neuraxial technique, and only one case of permanent injury was reported after peripheral nerve block among 16 studies.[6] In a review of 6,048 obstetric patients with nerve injuries, 93% of symptoms resolved in 6 months.[11] Including all anesthetic techniques, the recovery profile appears to be not as promising. In a study that included multiple anesthetic techniques for total joint arthroplasties with nerve injuries, 50–62% patients had complete neurologic recovery within 2 years, and 95–98% had complete or partial recovery overall.[12,13] Nerve injury due to tourniquets and peroneal and tibial nerve palsies after orthopedic cases have an overall good recovery profile, reported at 89–100% and 100%, respectively.[19] Ulnar nerve injuries have been well studied. After mean follow-up at 6 months, 47% patients still had symptoms; after 3 years, greater than one third of the patients remained symptomatic.[20] Motor deficits, particularly with lithotomy position, appear to have a worse recovery profile. In one of the largest retrospective studies with the longest follow-up, Warner et al.[7] followed patients who were in the lithotomy position with motor deficits, and "more than one half of the patients with a motor deficit at 3 months continued to have that deficit at 1 year, and one third of these patients who survived their procedure for at least 5 years continued to have the same deficit."

RISK FACTORS

ANESTHETIC TECHNIQUE

When counseling patients about risks of anesthetic care, anesthesiologists tend to include nerve injury in their disclaimer with peripheral nerve blocks and central neuraxial anesthetic, but not necessarily with general anesthesia or sedation cases. However, *all* techniques can lead to injury. Nerve injury is well known as a complication of neuraxial and non-neuraxial regional anesthesia (from needle or catheter-induced mechanical trauma), the neurotoxicity of injected drugs (mainly local anesthetics), and the blunting of protective reflexes within an anesthetized extremity.[21] For example, with epidurals and peripheral nerve catheter infusions, sensory block can delay diagnosis of neuropathies that have developed intraoperatively or are developing with certain casting and compressive devices. In addition, the motor block could allow the leg to be in positions that improperly stretch the nerves in therapy and movement. These risks call for enhanced awareness and patient monitoring with regional anesthesia techniques but should not preclude their use. Unfortunately, even with appropriate care and monitoring, nerve injuries still happen and it is often impossible to determine the cause. With general anesthesia, the mechanism of injury is less clear and possibly multifactorial, involving surgical manipulation (e.g., tourniquet, postoperative casting) and positioning, a presumed shared responsibility of surgeons, anesthesiologists, and other operating room staff.

There have been no prospective, randomized trials comparing neurologic outcomes between general and regional anesthesia. Given the rarity of the outcome, it is unlikely that this type of study will be conducted in a prospective fashion. As such, one must make inferences based on the existing data. General anesthesia was used in 86% of the ASA Closed-Claims Database cases with ulnar nerve injuries; the rest were a combination of regional or local anesthetic. Given the nature of the database, controls were not available.[1,2] The incidence of nerve injury with neuraxial anesthesia has been descrbied by some studies.[6,10] As was previously noted, however, multivariate analyses of nerve injury following total knee and hip arthroplasty did not find regional anesthesia to be predictive.[12,13] While nerve blocks were not associated with nerve injury, patients who underwent a nerve block and developed neurologic sequelae were less likely to fully recover. Despite being safe in limited doses and volumes, local anesthetics have a dose-dependent neurotoxicity and myotoxicity. Although not recommended by the American Society of Regional Anesthesia and Pain Medicine,[22] there is a small movement toward intentional intraneural injection, the rationale being that small volumes injected below the epineurium but outside the fascicles are safe.[23] Subepineural, extrafascicular injection may be easier in larger, more distal nerves, as they tend to have a higher ratio of connective tissue. It is hard to believe that clinicians can adequately distinguish intra- versus extra-fascicular injection within the nerve using even the highest-fidelity ultrasound available. Animal studies clearly demonstrate that neuropathy can be induced through needle damage, local anesthetics (especially when epinephrine is added), and high-pressure intraneural injection.[24,25]

Monitored anesthesia care appears to be protective against nerve injury, as the incidence is lower than that with other anesthestic techniques.[7,9,10] It is hypothesized that conscious patients retain more of their protective reflexes and are able to reposition themselves if injury and, presumably accompanying pain, occur. Increasing depth of sedation, longer anesthetics, and perioperative positioning can vary in monitored anesthesia care and may affect any potential protective effects.

PATIENT RISK FACTORS

On the basis of suspected pathophysiology of nerve injury and known risk factors of chronic neuropathy in nonsurgical patients, a number of risk factors have been studied using a variety of methods. An established patient risk factor for neuropathy is a pre-existing nerve injury, which can be subclinical or clinical. Alvine and Shurrer studied unilateral ulnar nerve palsies after general anesthesia, showing that 12 out of 14 patients had bilateral nerve conduction abnormalities.[20] Thus, if nerve function is already impaired at one location, this leaves the nerve more susceptible to injury at the same or another location along the same nerve. In nonsurgical patients, Upton and McComas attempted to explain impulse conduction abnormalities in the medial nerve, distal to the carpal tunnel, as well as surgical failure to improve carpal tunnel syndrome.[26] They proposed a "double crush" syndrome, showing that "most patients with carpal tunnel syndromes or ulnar neuropathies not only have compressive lesions at the wrist or elbows, but they have evidence of damage at the level of the cervical roots" (Figure 10.1).[26]

Normally, chemical substances are transmitted down the axon and secreted along the neuron; sensory receptors and downstream muscle fibers rely on this process. An injury that leads to a disruption of that supply will lead to symptoms. If an axon is already damaged, symptoms can be more severe than a comparable insult in a healthy nerve. Per EMG studies, it appears that "less compression of a median nerve at the carpal tunnel level … is required to produce symptoms when a cervical lesion is present."[27] In a more recent review of peroneal nerve palsies after total knee arthroplasty, patients with pre-existing neuropathies were at increased risk.[19] Perioperative nerve injuries in patients with pre-existing neurologic dysfunction are generally associated with poor outcomes.

Other patient risk factors that have been implicated are lower preoperative systolic blood pressure in orthopedic

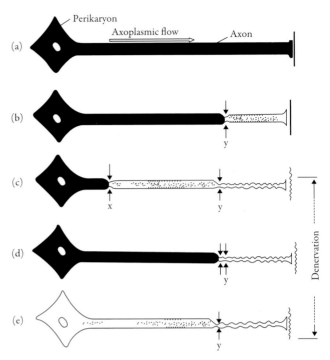

Figure 10.1 Displayed here are different types of neural lesions that can lead to denervation. Axoplasmic material is represented by the density of the shading. In a totally healthy neuron (**a**), axonal flow is complete. In a healthy neuron with one area of mild compression, flow is maintained distal to y (**b**). In a healthy neuron with two mild compressions (**c**), disruption of flow and thus denervation occurs distal to y, the point of compression. In a healthy neuron with severe compression (**d**), denervation also occurs distal to y. In an already compromised, sick neuron, such as in diabetes (**e**), one mild compression leads to denervation as the flow is already reduce proximal to y and continues to be further reduced distal to y. The essence of Upton's hypothesis is that impaired axoplasmic flow leads to denervation, instead of disrupted impulse conduction FROM UPTON AR, McComas AJ. The double crush in nerve entrapment syndromes. *Lancet* 1973;2(7825):359–362.

patients[19] and hypertension.[10] Hypertension is a disease that chronically affects blood flow—including the vaso vasorum, a blood supply network in peripheral nerves that is integral to the mechanism of injury. Furthermore, hypertensive patients, as well as patients with low preoperative blood pressure, could be more susceptible to hemodynamic instability and have associated pre-existing comorbidities that could affect outcome.

Most reviews of suspected patient risk factors in large studies have had mixed outcomes. Diabetes mellitus, a known cause of chronic neuropathy and vascular disease, has been shown to lead to an increased risk of incidence in studies with a wide variety of patient populations,[7,9,10] but not in orthopedic patients.[19] Tobacco use has been associated with an increased risk of nerve injury in a study of lithotomy position,[7] a large, retrospective review of all types of nerve injuries and anesthetics,[10] but not in two other trials of lithotomy position[8] and ulnar nerve injury.[9]

It is theorized that overweight or underweight patients are more likely to have nerve injury. Overweight patients are more difficult to position with standard operating room equipment, whereas underweight patients might have peripheral nerves that are less cushioned by protective body fat or tissue. However, results from studies of body mass index and nerve injury have been mixed: depending on the patient population, some studies have shown an association of injury with being obese or underweight, while others have shown no association at all.[7–9]

Most studies have shown no association of nerve injury with gender, with a few exceptions. Men appear more likely to incur ulnar neuropathy (70% men)[9] and brachial plexus injury in cardiac surgery, possibly due to a more shallow cubital tunnel.[28] Women have more injuries with total hip arthroplasties,[13] possible because of the higher prevalence of developmental hip dysplasia in women. Finally, increasing age has been associated with an increased risk of nerve injury in a variety of populations, including orthopedic and obstetric patients, as well as those underging surgery in lithotomy position.[7,11,19] However, other evaluations have shown no influence of age,[8,11] and yet others found associations of injury with younger ages,[13,19] possibly related to lower preoperative blood pressure.

INTRAOPERATIVE FACTORS

A variety of intraoperative factors have been proposed and studied. Longer anesthetic time has consistently been shown to increase risk.[11,13] In a large prospective study of postoperative motor neuropathy in almost a million patients from the National Surgical Quality Improvement Program (NSQIP) Database, Brummett et al.[29] found that an anesthetic time over 2 hours increased the risk of injury 4.4-fold, and an anesthetic time over 6 hours increased the risk 15.7-fold. Theoretically, the nerve is exposed to a longer duration of stretching and compression (leading to more ischemia and more severe injury), multiple positions, and possibly more perioperative bleeding and associated transfusions.[30] Hypotension and hypothermia have been proposed as risk factors of nerve injury, due to decreased blood flow, but these factors have been robustly studied only in cardiac surgery.

Intraoperative positioning has long been a focus of the anesthesiologist, as it is thought that avoidance of certain positions and appropriate padding can help prevent postoperative neuropathies. In a large, prospective evaluation of laboring patients, Wong et al.[11] found that a prolonged second stage of labor and a longer time pushing in the semi-Fowler-lithotomy positions were independent predictors of lower extremity injury. Another study found that each hour more in the lithotomy position increased the risk of neuropathy nearly 100-fold.[7] While padding the elbows to protect the ulnar nerve has become a part of standard anesthesia practice, one study found that patients who are hospitalized longer have a higher risk of nerve injury, particularly of the ulnar nerve.[31] This could occur from other confounding factors, such as a longer anesthetic time, or it could simply be that even medical patients develop ulnar nerve injury while in the hospital, likely from immobility.

Tourniquet time—specifically total time, longest interval without deflation, and least duration of deflation—is associated with a higher risk of nerve injury, likely from a combination of ischemia and mechanical trauma.[12,19] Each 30-minute increase in tourniquet inflation leads to a 3-fold risk in neurologic complications.

Certain surgeries have been presumed to be associated with a higher risk of nerve injury because they involve longer time in particular positions, surgical equipment more likely to induce injury, more potential blood loss and hemodynamic instability, and sicker patient populations. Patients undergoing cardiac surgery seem to have a higher incidence of nerve injury, especially to the ulnar nerve and brachial plexus.[28] Potential reasons for increased risk of nerve injury during cardiac surgery include sternal retraction, internal mammary artery dissection, internal jugular vein cannulation, pre-existing patient factors, and possibly hypothermia, length of case, and hemodynamic changes.[32] Obstetric patients also have a number of unique factors that may lead to perioperative nerve injury, such as pre-existing nerve damage from the ongoing pregnancy, intrinsic obstetric palsy, pushing in stirrups, assisted deliveries, and surgical retractors with caesarean sections.[11] Direct trauma during regional anesthesia is extremely rare. The presence of regional anesthesia can in theory increase the risk of nerve injury by prolonging the second stage of labor (a known risk factor for injury in itself) but has not been adequately studied.

Two studies compared multiple surgical subspecialties, finding a higher incidence of nerve injury with cardiac surgery, neurosurgery, and general surgery in one,[10] and spine, nonspine orthopedic, major vascular, and gynecologic surgery in the other.[29] Discrepancies between the two studies are likely due to the fact that one study investigated both sensory and motor neuropathies[10] and the other studied only motor injuries.[29] Although the exact mechanisms beyond this association are unclear, these surgeries might lead to a higher risk of nerve injury due to longer duration or prone positioning. As such, it may be worthwhile to discuss this increased risk with patients.

PREVENTIVE STRATEGIES AND TREATMENT

When a perioperative peripheral nerve injury occurs, the mechanism is often multifactorial or unclear. Thus, forming definite preventive strategies is difficult. Surgical causes of postoperative neuropathy are usually easier to define and can often be prevented with appropriate technique and monitoring. These include both intraoperative events (direct injury to the nerve, stretching of the nerve by the surgeon, long tourniquet time) and postoperative events (casting, crutches, compressive injuries, long postoperative admissions with immobility). It is recommended that tourniquet use be limited to 1–2 hours, as total tourniquet time is directly correlated with neuropathy.[19] Reperfusion has been advocated as a technique to extend the total duration of tourniquet time, but this has not been proven in human studies. Various tables and positions in orthopedic surgery have been studied, and their use in clinical care has been questioned.[13,19] Given the reported high incidence of neuropathy in the cardiac surgery population, expert recommendations have been made, including precise midline sternotomy to avoid asymmetric retraction, more caudal placement of retractors, and maintenance of neutral head position.[32] Regarding postoperative care, it is prudent to assess neurologic symptoms of patients daily. Neuropathy is most likely to present on the day of surgery or the first postoperative day[9,19,29] and should be immediately evaluated to ensure that there is no ongoing injury, such as a compartment syndrome, compression from a tight cast, or a compressive hematoma. Surgeons and internists caring for patients postoperatively should assess for new or ongoing symptoms; Warner et al.[31] showed that ulnar nerve injury occurs with nearly equal frequency in medical and surgical patients hospitalized for more than 2 days. Guidelines for postoperative follow-up are further expounded on in the ASA practice guidelines.[33]

It has been suggested that proper positioning and padding can prevent or decrease injury, but there have been no definitive data suggesting that certain intraoperative care patterns lead to fewer nerve injuries. Thus, it has become more commonly accepted that even the recommended methods of positioning and padding may not completely protect against injury in the most susceptible patients. In fact, in the ASA closed-claims review, 76% of the claims were judged by the reviewers to meet the standard of care for ulnar nerve injuries, while only 25% of the claims had documentation that the anesthetic provider placed extra padding over the elbows.[1] Thus, there is resistance to attributing ulnar neuropathy to improper positioning and padding. Interestingly, 63% of all nerve injury cases in the ASA Closed-Claims Database were judged to have met anesthetic standard of care, nearly twice the percentage of non-nerve claim cases. The ASA guidelines describe further preventive strategies.[33] Of course, limiting surgical and anesthetic time, especially in the lithotomy position, is warranted.

Whether regional anesthesia is associated with a higher incidence of neuropathy continues to be a point of controversy. As noted above, there are limited data comparing general to regional anesthesia. Regardless, recommendations to help prevent potential neuropathy for regional anesthesia have been made.[22] Whereas some recommend intentional intraneural/subepineural (but not intrafascicular) injection of small volumes of local anesthetic,[23] most experts recommend against this practice because of (1) the inability of clinicians to determine whether the subepineural injection is intra- or extra-fascicular and (2) the known neurotoxicity of intraneural or intrafascicular injections, especially with high pressure.[22,34] For peripheral nerve blocks, it is recommended that local anesthetic dose and volume be limited to that which is necessary to achieve a complete block. In addition, additives to local anesthetics should be limited to those that have been studied and deemed safe.[35]

TREATMENT OF POSTOPERATIVE NEUROPATHY

Symptoms and presentation dictate what treatment is necessary for perioperative peripheral nerve injuries. Most neuropathies are sensory in nature and manifest as numbness, paresthesias, and pain. Symptom management and time are normally all that is recommended for treatment, as most nerve injuries self-resolve.

Pain can be treated with anti-inflammatories, analgesics, or medications specifically for neuropathic pain, such as gabapentin.[4] Active use of the affected muscle is recommended, with physical therapy especially important to maintain range of motion after motor deficits. However, any further stress or traction on the nerve is discouraged, especially in immobilized patients, and compressive dressings should be removed.

Careful communication must occur between the surgical team and anesthesiologists to meet the goals of surgical recovery and further resolution of the nerve injury. Splints can also be used, with caution, to prevent further injuries to the damaged limb, but physical therapy should occur regularly for joint mobility. Surgical exploration is sometimes indicated for lesions that do not heal. However, waiting up

Table 10.1 RECOMMENDATIONS FOR POSITIONING TO REDUCE NEUROPATHIES, FROM THE ASA PRACTICE GUIDELINES FOR PREVENTION OF PERIOPERATIVE PERIPHERAL NERVE INJURY (2011)[33]

Upper extremities	Brachial plexus in a supine patient	Arm abduction limited to 90 degrees in a supine patient
	Brachial plexus in a prone patient	May allow abduction greater than 90 degrees comfortably
	Ulnar with arms on arm board	Arm positioning to decrease pressure on postcondylar groove of the humerus, either by supination or the neutral forearm position
	Ulnar with arms tucked at side	Arms should be in a neutral position
	Ulnar with flexion of the elbow	May increase risk of neuropathy, but no acceptable degree stated
	Radial	Prolonged pressure on the radial nerve in the spiral groove of the humerus should be avoided
	Median	Extension of the elbow beyond the range that is comfortable during the preoperative assessment
Lower extremities	Sciatic	Stretching of the hamstring muscle group beyond the range that is comfortable during preoperative assessment may stretch the nerve
	Sciatic	Extension and flexion of the hips and knee joints should be considered when determining degree of flexion, as sciatic nerve crosses both
	Femoral	Neither flexion or extension increases the risk of neuropathy.
	Peroneal	Prolonged pressure on the peroneal nerve at the fibular head should be avoided
Protective padding	Arm boards, chest rolls, padding at the elbow, padding to protect the peroneal nerve	All may decrease the risk of neuropathies
	Inappropriately used, i.e., too tight, padding	May increase the risk of neuropathies
Equipment	Properly functioning automated blood pressure cuff, i.e., above antecubital fossa	Does not seem to change the risk of upper extremity neuropathy
	The use of shoulder braces in a steep head down position	May increase the risk of neuropathies
Documentation	May be useful to focus attention on positioning	
	Provide information on strategies that leads to improvement in patient care	
Postoperative assessment	A simple evaluation of extremity nerve function may lead to early recognition of peripheral neuropathies	

to a year for signs of recovery is recommended prior to any surgery . Neurolysis can be performed for pain control but is not always effective and can potentially worsen painful symptoms.

Other methods include resection and grafting of non-conducting lesions and transposition of nerves. Dorsal column and peripheral nerve stimulation may provide some benefit in refractory cases; however, there are no data for this treatment in postoperative neuropathy patients.

CURRENT GUIDELINES AND RECOMMENDATIONS

Despite years of research, the mechanisms driving periop-erative neuropathy are still not fully elucidated. It is well accepted that perioperative neuropathies sometimes occur despite appropriate positioning and padding of the limbs during surgery. As most studies are retrospective in nature and nerve injuries are rare, there have been few prospective studies investigating preventative techniques or the impact of various positioning and padding techniques. Therefore, guidelines are based on expert recommendations. The ASA practice advisory for the prevention of perioperative peripheral nerve injury released updated recommendations in 2011, focusing on "the perioperative positioning of the adult patient, use of protective padding, and the avoid-ance of contact with hard surfaces or supports that may apply direct pressure on susceptible peripheral nerves."[33] It also recommends that patients be evaluated preoperatively regarding the positions they can tolerate tolerated during surgery. Any limitations to range of motion expected in the operating room should be reviewed with the surgeons and nursing staff. Furthermore, patients should be counseled preoperatively of their increased risk of injury. A survey of surgical patients indicated that patients would like the risk of nerve palsy discussed prior to the operation.[36] Key portions of the ASA guidelines are noted in Table 10.1. The American Society of Regional Anesthesia and Pain Medicine has also authored a practice advisory on neurologic complications from regional anesthesia in 2008, and an update is expected in 2013.[22]

There are no data available to help clinicians determine the risks and benefits of general versus regional anesthesia with respect to the potential for postoperative neuropathy. There are benefits to regional anesthesia, such as avoidance of opioid-induced side effects and improved pain relief, which may outweigh any additional risk of nerve injury. Regional anesthesia is not recommended in patients with known disorders of the central and peripheral nervous systems, such as multiple sclerosis, diabetic neuropathy, and chemotherapy-induced neuropathy. Except for pediatric patients and rare situations, regional anesthesia is not recommended in patients that are deeply anesthetized or deeply sedated, as this prevents patients from reporting symptoms during the procedure.[22] Only local anesthetics and adjuvants with demonstrated safety profiles should be used.[35] Conventional wisdom on the required dose and volume of local anesthetic required to conduct a peripheral nerve block has been challenged in recent years.[37] Since local anesthetics have a dose- and time-dependent neurotoxic effect, consideration of the minimum amount of local anesthetic required is recommended. Although these guidelines are intended to aid the anesthesiologist and patient in medical decision making, the risks and benefits must always be considered at the level of the individual patient.

The ASA practice advisory specifically suggests a focused history and physical examination to identify patients with certain pre-existing risk factors. As described above, patient risk factors likely constitute much of the unexplained variance seen in perioperative neuropathy outcomes; however, other factors, including the duration of surgery and intraoperative positioning, must be included. Given the low incidence of nerve injury, it is almost impossible to predict this outcome, and patients should simply be informed that they may be at higher risk. Patients at increased risk for nerve injury due to comorbidities or high-risk surgery are also likely at risk for other adverse perioperative outcomes, including myocardial infarction, stroke and renal failure. Despite clearly being a common reason for filing claims against anesthesiologists as listed in the ASA closed-claims data,[1,2] the perceived severity of nerve injury,

when compared to other serious potential outcomes, make it unlikely to be the primary concern of patients preoperatively. Anesthesiologists and surgeons must, however, consider the risk in their perioperative planning.

Intraoperatively, the ASA practice advisory explores a variety of considerations for each stated position, but the experts clearly admit to the paucity of data driving these recommendations. Regarding the upper extremities, there are no data regarding means of preventing radial or median neuropathies. For brachial plexus protection, experts recommend limiting abduction of the arm to 90 degrees in a supine patient. For ulnar nerve protection, one should avoid prolonged flexion, ensure that there is no pressure on the ulnar groove when using an arm board, and tuck the arm in neutral position. For the lower extremities, one should limit hip flexion and limit knee extension in order to protect the sciatic nerve as it crosses these joints. Also, reducing pressure on the peroneal nerve at the fibular head is advised, especially in the lithotomy position. These recommendations are based on anatomic reasons and case reports. Regarding protective padding, only case studies exist. The ASA practice advisory states that "padded arm boards, chest rolls in the lateral position, padding at the elbow, padding at the fibular head ... may decrease the risk of neuropathy."[33] There is no consensus as to whether automated blood pressure cuffs increase the risk of any neuropathy. Shoulder braces "may increase the risk of perioperative neuropathies" in the steep head-down position.

Finally, there should be a postoperative assessment to identify peripheral neuropathies. The great majority (66–86%) of perioperative peripheral nerve injuries are noted on postoperative day 0 or 1,[19,29] but some do not develop symptoms until 2–7 days after the surgery.[9] Inpatients should be routinely questioned by anesthesiologists about any new neurologic symptoms, and outpatients should be asked in postoperative phone interviews specifically about nerve injury symptoms.

Earlier detection of these injuries, especially with motor symptoms, can lead to full evaluations by a neurologist. First, the new symptoms and findings should be distinguished from other afflictions,[4] including cervical spine injuries, other musculoskeletal disorders, and autoimmune neurologic disorders. Electromyography can also be performed. It is critical to evaluate for ongoing and modifiable neuropathies, as would be seen with tight casts and compartment syndromes. One disorder that can present postoperatively, unrelated to any direct intraoperative mechanism, is acute brachial plexitis: an inflammatory disorder of the brachial plexus that is related to the stress of surgery.[38] It persists with severe shoulder pain, radiating down the arm, lasting hours to weeks, and is a diagnosis of exclusion. Finally, proper documentation should occur, something that has been proven to be inadequate.

CONCLUSIONS

Neuropathy is a rare but potentially devastating complication of surgery and anesthesia. Studies have demonstrated some of the patient, anesthetic, and surgical factors associated with perioperative nerve injury. Despite the large number of patients included in some of the prospective and retrospective studies, there are no datasets available at this time that adequately address the various risk factors in such a way as to better understand the wide variance seen in outcomes. More studies including patient comorbidities, detailed anesthetic records, patient positioning, surgical data, and structured postoperative neurologic assessments are needed. In the meantime, clinicians should follow the expert recommendations detailed in the available practice advisories.[22,33]

CONFLICT OF INTEREST STATEMENT

C.B.: The University of Michigan has filed for a patent application covering the use of dexmedetomidine alone and as an additive to local anesthetic to enhance efficacy and safety in peripheral nerve blockade. Brummett CM, Inventor; The Regents of the University of Michigan, Assignee; Anesthetic Methods and Compositions; US patent application US 12/791,506; June 1, 2010. C.B. has no other conflicts of interest or financial disclosures.

M.B.W. has no conflicts of interest to disclose

REFERENCES

1. Cheney FW, Domino KB, Caplan RA, Posner KL. Nerve injury associated with anesthesia: a closed claims analysis. *Anesthesiology.* 1999;90(4):1062–1069.
2. Kroll DA, Caplan RA, Posner K, Ward RJ, Cheney FW. Nerve injury associated with anesthesia. *Anesthesiology.* 1990;73(2):202–207.
3. Prielipp RC, Morell RC, Butterworth J. Ulnar nerve injury and perioperative arm positioning. *Anesthesiol Clin North Am.* 2002;20(3):589–603.
4. Winfree CJ, Kline DG. Intraoperative positioning nerve injuries. *Surg Neurol.* 2005;63(1):5–18.
5. Seddon HJ. Three types of nerve injury. *Brain.* 1942;66:237.
6. Brull R, McCartney CJ, Chan VW, El-Beheiry H. Neurological complications after regional anesthesia: contemporary estimates of risk. *Anesth Analg.* 2007;104(4):965–974.
7. Warner MA, Martin JT, Schroeder DR, Offord KP, Chute CG. Lower-extremity motor neuropathy associated with surgery performed on patients in a lithotomy position. *Anesthesiology.* 1994;81(1):6–12.
8. Warner MA, Warner DO, Harper CM, Schroeder DR, Maxson PM. Lower extremity neuropathies associated with lithotomy positions. *Anesthesiology.* 2000;93(4):938–942.
9. Warner MA, Warner ME, Martin JT. Ulnar neuropathy. Incidence, outcome, and risk factors in sedated or anesthetized patients. *Anesthesiology.* 1994;81(6):1332–1340.
10. Welch MB, Brummett CM, Welch TD, et al. Perioperative peripheral nerve injuries: a retrospective study of 380,680 cases during a 10-year period at a single institution. *Anesthesiology.* 2009;111(3):490–497.
11. Wong CA, Scavone BM, Dugan S, et al. Incidence of postpartum lumbosacral spine and lower extremity nerve injuries. *Obstet Gynecol.* 2003;101(2):279–288.
12. Jacob AK, Mantilla CB, Sviggum HP, Schroeder DR, Pagnano MW, Hebl JR. Perioperative nerve injury after total knee arthroplasty: regional anesthesia risk during a 20-year cohort study. *Anesthesiology.* 2011;114(2):311–317.
13. Jacob AK, Mantilla CB, Sviggum HP, Schroeder DR, Pagnano MW, Hebl JR. Perioperative nerve injury after total hip arthroplasty: regional anesthesia risk during a 20-year cohort study. *Anesthesiology.* 2011;115(6):1172–1178.
14. Auroy Y, Benhamou D, Bargues L, et al. Major complications of regional anesthesia in France: the SOS Regional Anesthesia Hotline Service. *Anesthesiology.* 2002;97(5):1274–1280.
15. Borgeat A, Ekatodramis G, Kalberer F, Benz C. Acute and nonacute complications associated with interscalene block and shoulder surgery: a prospective study. *Anesthesiology.* 2001;95(4):875–880.
16. Candido KD, Sukhani R, Doty R, Jr., et al. Neurologic sequelae after interscalene brachial plexus block for shoulder/upper arm surgery: the association of patient, anesthetic, and surgical factors to the incidence and clinical course. *Anesth Analg.* 2005;100(5):1489–1495.
17. Liu SS, Zayas VM, Gordon MA, et al. A prospective, randomized, controlled trial comparing ultrasound versus nerve stimulator guidance for interscalene block for ambulatory shoulder surgery for postoperative neurological symptoms. *Anesth Analg.* 2009;109(1):265–271.
18. Capdevila X, Pirat P, Bringuier S, et al. Continuous peripheral nerve blocks in hospital wards after orthopedic surgery: a multicenter prospective analysis of the quality of postoperative analgesia and complications in 1,416 patients. *Anesthesiology.* 2005;103(5):1035–1045.
19. Horlocker TT, Hebl JR, Gali B, et al. Anesthetic, patient, and surgical risk factors for neurologic complications after prolonged total tourniquet time during total knee arthroplasty. *Anesth Analg.* 2006;102(3):950–955.
20. Alvine FG, Schurrer ME. Postoperative ulnar-nerve palsy. Are there predisposing factors? *J Bone Joint Surg Am.* 1987;69(2):255–259.
21. Hogan QH. Pathophysiology of peripheral nerve injury during regional anesthesia. *Reg Anesth Pain Med.* 2008;33(5):435–441.
22. Neal JM, Bernards CM, Hadzic A, et al. ASRA practice advisory on neurologic complications in regional anesthesia and pain medicine. *Reg Anesth Pain Med.* 2008;33(5):404–415.
23. Bigeleisen PE. Nerve puncture and apparent intraneural injection during ultrasound-guided axillary block does not invariably result in neurologic injury. *Anesthesiology.* 2006;105(4):779–783.
24. Selander D, Brattsand R, Lundborg G, Nordborg C, Olsson Y. Local anesthetics: importance of mode of application, concentration and adrenaline for the appearance of nerve lesions. An experimental study of axonal degeneration and barrier damage after intrafascicular injection or topical application of bupivacaine (Marcain). *Acta Anaesthesiol Scand.* 1979;23(2):127–136.
25. Hadzic A, Dilberovic F, Shah S, et al. Combination of intraneural injection and high injection pressure leads to fascicular injury and neurologic deficits in dogs. *Reg Anesth Pain Med.* 2004;29(5):417–423.
26. Upton AR, McComas AJ. The double crush in nerve entrapment syndromes. *Lancet.* 1973;2(7825):359–362.
27. Osterman AL. The double crush syndrome. *Orthop Clin North Am.* 1988;19(1):147–155.

28. Lederman RJ, Breuer AC, Hanson MR, et al. Peripheral nervous system complications of coronary artery bypass graft surgery. *Ann Neurol.* 1982;12(3):297–301.

29. Brummett CM, Mashour GA, Shanks AM, Welch MB, Kheterpal S. Preoperative and intraoperative risk factors for acute postoperative motor neuropathy. Paper presented at: American Society of Anesthesiologists Annual Meeting; October 18, 2010.

30. Horlocker TT, Cabanela ME, Wedel DJ. Does postoperative epidural analgesia increase the risk of peroneal nerve palsy after total knee arthroplasty? *Anesth Analg.* 1994;79(3):495–500.

31. Warner MA, Warner DO, Harper CM, Schroeder DR, Maxson PM. Ulnar neuropathy in medical patients. *Anesthesiology.* 2000;92(2):613–615.

32. Sharma AD, Parmley CL, Sreeram G, Grocott HP. Peripheral nerve injuries during cardiac surgery: risk factors, diagnosis, prognosis, and prevention. *Anesth Analg.* 2000;91(6):1358–1369.

33. Practice advisory for the prevention of perioperative peripheral neuropathies: an updated report by the American Society of Anesthesiologists Task Force on prevention of perioperative peripheral neuropathies. *Anesthesiology.* 2011;114(4):741–754.

34. Selander D. Neurotoxicity of local anesthetics: animal data. *Reg Anesth.* 1993;18(6 Suppl):461–468.

35. Brummett CM, Williams BA. Additives to local anesthetics for peripheral nerve blockade. *Int Anesthesiol Clin.* 2011;49(4):104–116.

36. Ek ET, Yu EP, Chan JT, Love BR. Nerve injuries in orthopaedics: is there anything more we need to tell our patients? *ANZ J Surg.* 2005;75(3):132–135.

37. Riazi S, Carmichael N, Awad I, Holtby RM, McCartney CJ. Effect of local anaesthetic volume (20 vs 5 ml) on the efficacy and respiratory consequences of ultrasound-guided interscalene brachial plexus block. *Br J Anaesth.* 2008;101(4):549–556.

38. Griffin AC, Wood WG. Brachial plexitis: a rare and often misdiagnosed postoperative complication. *Aesthetic Plast Surg.* 1996;20(3):263–265.

11.

POSTOPERATIVE VISUAL LOSS AND ISCHEMIC OPTIC NEUROPATHY

Vijay Kumar Ramaiah and Lorri A. Lee

INTRODUCTION

Partial or complete loss of vision in the perioperative period is a devastating iatrogenic complication that can leave patients with significant physical disability and loss of quality of life. Postoperative visual loss (POVL) with nonocular surgery most often occurs in association with cardiac surgery, spine surgery in the prone position, and head and neck surgery.[1] POVL has also been reported in other operations, including nonspine orthopedic surgery, major vascular surgery, prostatectomies (open or laparoscopic/robotic), abdominal compartment syndrome, liposuction, thoracotomies, liver transplantation, and other miscellaneous cases.

The four most common POVL diagnoses are central retinal artery occlusion (CRAO), cortical blindness, anterior ischemic optic neuropathy (AION), and posterior ischemic optic neuropathy (PION). Less common POVL diagnoses include glycine toxicity during transurethral resection of the prostate (TURP), acute angle closure glaucoma, expansion of intraocular gas perfluoropropane (C3F8) and sulfur hexafluoride (SF6) with administration of nitrous oxide containing anesthetics, and posterior reversible encephalopathic syndrome (PRES).[2–6] This chapter will focus on the more common types of POVL, with an emphasis on AION and PION.

BACKGROUND
ANATOMY AND BLOOD SUPPLY OF THE OPTIC NERVE AND RETINA

The blood supply to the optic nerve varies from the retina to the optic nerve head, to the intraorbrtal optic nerve, the intracanalicular optic nerve, the intracranial optic nerve, the chiasm, the optic tracts, and to the occipital cortex. Numerous variations exist, and the most common patterns of vasculature will be discussed herein. The retina is supplied primarily from the central retinal artery, originating from the ophthalmic artery approximately 10 to 12 mm posterior to the globe and coursing through the center of the nerve to the retina.[7] It splits into four major branches supplying the four quadrants of the retina. Additional retinal blood flow comes from the choroidal circulation from the short posterior ciliary arteries, which also arise from the ophthalmic artery. The choroidal circulation is the predominant blood supply to the macula.

The optic nerve head is supplied by the central retinal artery and the short posterior ciliary arteries, but with a greater contribution from the ciliary arteries. Posterior ciliary artery branches anastomose to make up the circle of Zinn-Haller that perfuses the optic nerve head. Recurrent choroidal arterioles and recurrent pial arterioles also contribute to the optic nerve head blood supply and arise

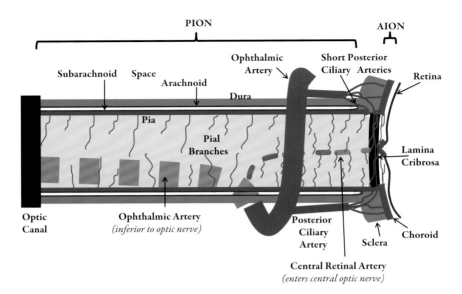

Figure 11.1 Diagram of the orbital portion of the optic nerve. The ophthalmic artery supplies the orbital optic nerve via the posterior ciliary arteries (and choroidal arteries), the central retinal artery, numerous direct branches to the optic nerve, and the fine pial vasculature supplied by these vessels that surround the orbital portion of the optic nerve. Note the watershed zone in the posterior portion of the central orbital nerve where there are minimal centrifugal pial vessels in the center of the optic nerve. PION, posterior ischemic optic neuropathy With permission from Lee LA, Mudumbai R. Postoperative visual loss. In *Anesthesia for Spine Surgery*. Cambridge University Press, New York. 2012. Fig. 15.1, p. 259. Illustration by Lorri A. Lee, M.D., University of Washington, Seattle, WA.

from the posterior ciliary arteries. Branches from the short posterior ciliary arteries that supply the optic nerve head have nonfenestrated endothelial cells with tight junctions encompassed by pericytes, thus creating an effective blood–brain, or blood–nerve barrier. Gadolinium enhancement on magnetic resonance imaging will not be visible unless this barrier is damaged.[7] The prelaminar portion of the optic nerve may have less "tight" capillary junctions than those of the retina or the remainder of the optic nerve.[8] Similar to intracranial blood vessels, the optic nerve head vasculature is able to autoregulate to maintain relatively stable blood flow over a range of intraocular and systemic pressures.[7] Likewise, there is considerable variation between individuals in the extent of autoregulation in the optic nerve head.[9]

The optic nerve and optic chiasm are supplied through a continuous overlying pial plexus.[10] The pial circulation of the intraorbital part of optic nerve is supplied either directly from small ophthalmic artery branches or from recurrent short posterior ciliary and central retinal arteries, both of which arise from the ophthalmic artery (Figure 11.1). Both centrifugal and centripetal pial vessels supply the portion of the optic nerve through which the central retinal artery runs. Posterior to where the central retinal artery pierces the optic nerve, only the centripetal pial vessels penetrate the optic nerve, rendering the central optic nerve potentially more susceptible to hypoperfusion.

The intracanalicular part of the optic nerve receives blood flow from small branches of the ophthalmic artery arising just distal to the optic canal, namely the medial collateral, lateral collateral, and ventral branches.[7] These branches supply the pial surface and then penetrate the optic nerve. Posterior to the optic canal, no dura or arachnoid surrounds the optic nerve. The intracranial part of the nerve and optic chiasm are fed by the internal carotid artery and branches including the anterior cerebral, anterior communicating, and superior hypophyseal artery. The posterior communicating artery may contribute branches to the posterior chiasm and is the main blood supply to the optic tracts along with the anterior choroidal arteries.[7] The retrogeniculate optic radiation and occipital cortex are supplied by the middle and posterior cerebral arteries.

The venous drainage of the orbit is not symmetric with the arterial vasculature and is valveless, similar to the other head and neck veins.[8] The majority of the venous outflow from the orbit is carried by the superior ophthalmic vein. The retina and anterior optic nerve empty into the central retinal vein, which drains into the superior ophthalmic vein. Choroidal venous flow travels through the vortex venous system that drains into the superior and inferior ophthalmic veins and ultimately into the cavernous sinus (Figure 11.2).

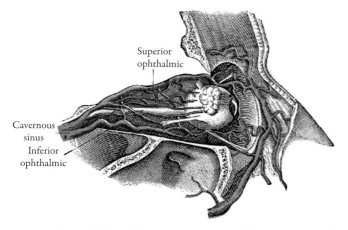

Superior
ophthalmic

Cavernous
sinus

Inferior
ophthalmic

Figure 11.2 Figure 572 from Henry Gray's *Anatomy of the Human Body* (1918) showing venous drainage of the orbit. The superior ophthalmic vein is the main venous outflow for the orbit. The retina and anterior optic nerve empty into the central retinal vein, which drains into the superior ophthalmic vein. Choroidal venous flow travels through the vortex venous system that drains into the superior and inferior ophthalmic veins and ultimately into the cavernous sinus.

MAJOR POVL DIAGNOSES AND OPHTHALMOLOGIC EXAMINATION

For any cases of POVL, an urgent ophthalmologic consultation should be obtained, preferably by a neuro-ophthalmologist, if available. Despite the poor prognosis for the four major types of POVL, other rare causes of POVL may be treatable, and specialists are more likely to be aware of any new advances in therapy. Before discussing etiology and prevention of ION, it is important to have a basic understanding of the ophthalmologic examination findings with the most common types of POVL to fully appreciate possible etiologies and prognosis. Computed tomography (CT) or magnetic resonance imaging (MRI) of the head may be useful to detect infarctions of the visual pathway or other catastrophic intracranial events. At this time, no reliable radiologic imaging is available for detecting acute injury of the optic nerve. Visual acuity and field testing, pupillary reflexes, and fundoscopic examination differ for each of the four major causes of POVL (Table 11.1).

Table 11.1 **MAJOR TYPES OF POSTOPERATIVE VISUAL LOSS: CLINICAL PRESENTATION, WORKUP, AND PROGNOSIS**

	CRAO	CORTICAL BLINDNESS	AION	PION
Most common procedures	Head and neck, spine, cardiac	Cardiac, thoracovascular, spine, nonfusion orthopedic	Cardiac, spine, nonfusion orthopedic, head and neck	Spine, head and neck, thoracovascular, cardiac
Timing of complaint after emergence from anesthesia and lucid	Immediate	Immediate; occasionally patient's may be unaware of their blindness	Immediate to several days postoperatively; may have normal vision initially	Immediate
Clinical course	No worsening; one third may have some recovery—rarely complete recovery	No worsening; more than half may recover—frequently complete recovery, though many left with deficits in spatial orientation	May progress for several days after onset; approximately one third with some recovery—rarely complete recovery	No worsening; approximately one third may have some recovery—rarely complete recovery
Unilateral vs. bilateral	Unilateral	Usually bilateral	Bilateral > unilateral	Bilateral >> unilateral
Visual Defects				
Visual field defects	Usually complete loss of vision in affected eye	Usually bilateral homonymous hemianopsia; if unilateral infarct (e.g., emboli), may have contralateral homonymous hemianopsia	Central scotoma, altitudinal field cuts, or complete loss of vision	Central scotoma, altitudinal field cuts, or complete loss of vision
Pupillary light reflex	Absent or sluggish with RAPD	Normal	Absent or sluggish with RAPD if defect is unilateral or asymmetric	Absent or sluggish with RAPD if defect is unilateral or asymmetric
Fundoscopic examination	EARLY: ischemic, pale, white retina; cherry red spot at macula LATE: may develop optic disc pallor; retina may reperfuse	EARLY: normal LATE: normal	EARLY: Optic disc edema; frequent peripapillary flame-shaped hemorrhages or splinter hemorrhages at optic disc margin. LATE: optic disc pallor	EARLY: normal. LATE: optic disc pallor
Computed tomography/ magnetic resonance imaging	Normal or may show extraocular muscle edema/damage from compression	Parieto-occipital infarctions—usually bilateral with occlusive or watershed infarctions—or punctuate with embolic infarctions	Usually normal, occasionally may show optic nerve edema	Usually normal, occasionally may show optic nerve edema

Supplementary confirmatory tests such as visual evoked potentials to detect optic nerve injury and electroretinogram to detect retinal ischemia may also be performed when patient cooperation is inadequate for the visual testing or diagnostic uncertainty is present.

CENTRAL RETINAL ARTERY OCCLUSION

CRAO interrupt blood supply to the retina (Figure 11.3A, normal fundus; and Figure 11.3B, CRAO), and is most commonly associated with prone spine surgery and procedures with high embolic loads, such as cardiac bypass.[11] Because the visual loss is typically unilateral and complete, patients will usually voice complaints shortly after emergence from anesthesia. Periorbital trauma such as bruising, erythema, swelling, proptosis, or ophthalmoplegia are frequently present when the injury is caused by globe compression in the perioperative setting.[12] Pupillary light reflexes are typically absent or sluggish with a relative afferent pupillary defect. Fundoscopic examination can be dramatic with ischemia or whitening of the entire retina, thin attenuated vessels, and a "cherry red spot" caused by the separate choriocapillaris blood supply to the macula, which is typically unaffected in this injury.[1] Electroretinograms are abnormal with an increased "a" wave and severely decreased or absent "b" wave.[13] No known beneficial treatment exists at this time for perioperative CRAO, and recovery of vision is poor.

CORTICAL BLINDNESS

Cortical blindness is typically caused by emboli to the parieto-occipital cortex or by profound hypoperfusion

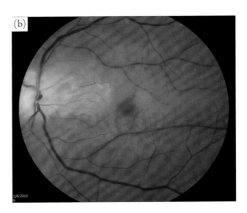

Figure 11.3b Central retinal artery occlusion (CRAO), resolving. Note both the whitened, pale, ischemic areas along with reperfused retina, and the cherry red spot at the macula. The cherry red spot is where the choriocapillaris supplies the macula With permission from Lee LA, Mudumbai R. Postoperative visual loss. In *Anesthesia for Spine Surgery*. Cambridge University Press, New York. 2012. Fig. 15.2A-D, p. 259–261. Photographs by Raghu Mudumbai, M.D., University of Washington, Seattle, WA.

with bilateral posterior watershed infarctions. It is most commonly associated with cardiac bypass procedures, spinal fusion surgery (especially in children), and nonfusion orthopedic procedures such as hip and knee replacement surgery.[11] Visual symptoms usually present when the patient first wakens or is lucid and can range from a contralateral homonymous hemianopsia, when the lesion is unilateral, to bilateral homonymous hemianopsia to bilateral complete loss of vision.[1] Occasionally, a small island of central vision may be spared with bilateral lesions. Pupillary light reflexes are intact and the fundoscopic examination is normal. Brain CT or MRI shows punctate occipital infarctions in the posterior cerebral artery territory, or parieto-occipital infarctions in a watershed distribution that are typically bilateral.[1] Unlike CRAO, AION, and PION, improvement of vision can be profound with cortical blindness, with dramatic improvement in the first few weeks. However, patients may have permanent defects in spatial orientation despite normal visual acuity and visual fields.[13]

ANTERIOR ISCHEMIC OPTIC NEUROPATHY

AION in the perioperative period is almost exclusively of the nonarteritic type and is sometimes referred to as nAION. Arteritic AION, most commonly known as temporal arteritis, is rarely found in the operative setting. Nonarteritic AION is much more common in the nonoperative setting where it can occur spontaneously.[1] In the nonsurgical population, it has been associated with risk factors for vaso-occlusive disease with presentation typically in the sixth decade of life or later. Nonarteritic AION in the

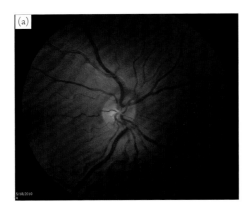

Figure 11.3a Normal fundus. Note the distinct optic disc margin with well-perfused retinal vessels and a pink retina. Posterior ischemic optic neuropathy appears entirely normal in the first weeks to months, prior to the development of optic nerve pallor. Cortical blindness also has a normal fundus With permission from Lee LA, Mudumbai R. Postoperative visual loss. In *Anesthesia for Spine Surgery*. Cambridge University Press, New York. 2012. Fig. 15.2A-D, p. 259–261. Photographs by Raghu Mudumbai, M.D., University of Washington, Seattle, WA.

nonoperative setting typically presents with unilateral partial loss of vision that progresses over several days or more. Its exact etiology and pathophysiologic mechanism remain unknown, and effective treatment has not been identified.

Perioperative AION is associated most commonly with cardiac bypass procedures, prone spine surgery, major vascular surgery, open prostatectomies, and a variety of miscellaneous procedures.[1,11,13] Patients may have symptoms on awakening from anesthesia; but unlike the other major types of POVL, the patient may have normal vision initially after surgery, with onset of progressive visual loss one to several days after surgery.[1] Visual symptoms are more commonly bilateral and more severe compared to those of AION in the nonoperative setting. Pupillary light reflexes may be absent to sluggish with a relative afferent pupillary defect if the defect is unilateral or asymmetric.[1] Visual field deficits can range from central scotoma to altitudinal field cuts to complete loss of vision. Fundoscopic examination reveals an edematous optic disk frequently with peripapillary flame-shaped hemorrhages or splinter hemorrhages at the optic disc margin (Figure 11.3C)[1]. Several weeks later, the swelling subsides and the heme gets reabsorbed as the optic disc turns pale (Figure 11.3D). At this late point, AION and PION may appear identical with optic nerve pallor. Visual evoked potentials will be abnormal with a depressed amplitude and near-normal latency or unidentifiable waveform.[13] Many treatments for perioperative AION have been attempted and will be detailed later in this chapter; however, none have proven consistently efficacious. Prognosis for visual recovery with perioperative AION is also poor, almost never returning to baseline vision.

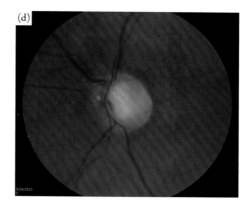

Figure 11.3d Optic nerve pallor. Once the ganglion cells have died, the optic disc becomes whitened With permission from Lee LA, Mudumbai R. Postoperative visual loss. In *Anesthesia for Spine Surgery*. Cambridge University Press, New York. 2012. Fig. 15.2A-D, p. 259–261. Photographs by Raghu Mudumbai, M.D., University of Washington, Seattle, WA.

POSTERIOR ISCHEMIC OPTIC NEUROPATHY

PION typically occurs in the setting of elevated venous pressure in the head with procedures such as prone spine surgery, bilateral radical head and neck surgery in the prone position, robotic/laparoscopic prostatectomies with the head in steep Trendelenburg position for prolonged duration, and a variety of miscellaneous cases.[1,12,13] Patients typically complain of visual loss on awakening from anesthesia, though complaints may be delayed if the patient is kept on mechanical ventilation overnight or is not fully lucid. POVL from PION is frequently severe with complete blindness; bilateral involvement is present in two thirds of cases.[12] Symptoms occasionally may be as mild as "blurry" vision with central scotoma or altitudinal field cuts in only one eye. Pupillary light reflexes are similar to those in AION, ranging from absent to sluggish with a relative afferent pupillary defect when the injury is unilateral or asymmetric.[1] Early fundoscopic examination is normal (Figure 11.3A) with progression to optic disc pallor over weeks to months (Figure 11.3D). Visual evoked potential and electroretinogram testing is similar to that for AION. Likewise, no proven beneficial treatments are known, and recovery from PION in the perioperative setting is very poor.

INCIDENCE AND PREVALENCE OF PERIOPERATIVE ISCHEMIC OPTIC NEUROPATHY

SINGLE AND MULTI-INSTITUTIONAL DATA

The incidence of POVL varies according to single- or multiple-institutional studies or national data, type of surgery examined, and definition of POVL. These studies are all limited by their retrospective design and/or use of

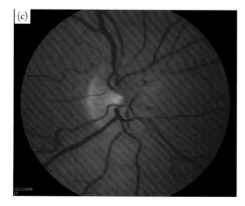

Figure 11.3c Anterior ischemic optic neuropathy (AION); early examination in AION where there is swelling at the superior right optic disc margin with peripapillary flame-shaped hemorrhages. After weeks to months, the swelling subsides, the heme is absorbed, and optic nerve pallor develops (see Figure 11.3d) With permission from Lee LA, Mudumbai R. Postoperative visual loss. In *Anesthesia for Spine Surgery*. Cambridge University Press, New York. 2012. Fig. 15.2A-D, p. 259–261. Photographs by Raghu Mudumbai, M.D., University of Washington, Seattle, WA.

billing data to identify cases of POVL. POVL incidence data from single institutions for all nonocular surgery have been reported as between 0.0008% and 0.0016%, whereas single-institutional data for spine surgery has been reported as between 0.028% and 0.09%, demonstrating a minimum 50-fold increase in incidence in spine surgery.[14–16] Stevens et al. documented the highest reported incidence for multi-institutional data at 0.2% for all causes of POVL after spine surgery and at 0.1% for ION.[17] Variations in incidence of POVL between institutions may reflect variations in patient populations, types of procedures performed, accuracy in diagnostic coding, and unkown perioperative practice variations.

NATIONAL DATA

The Nationwide Inpatient Sample (NIS) is the largest inpatient all-payer database in the United States containing discharge data from over 1000 randomly selected hospitals across the country. It is estimated to cover approximately 20% of community hospital discharges in the United States. Data collected in the NIS include demographics, specific diagnoses and procedures, hospital length of stay, hospital charges, and some outcome measures. This database is useful for studies involving demographics, charges, length of stay, some diagnoses, and procedures. Use of this database for assessment of risk factors for perioperative complications must be done with caution because significant bias may exist in the assessment of patients and collection of data between patients with and without complications. Entry of these data into the hospital discharge database is frequently done by billing personnel and its accuracy cannot be validated. Further, collection of potentially confounding data such as blood loss, operative duration, fluid administration, hemodynamics, specific surgical devices, and other intraoperative and postoperative details is poor. These data are more commonly used for health care utilization and cost-of-care studies.

Studies using the NIS database reported an overall incidence of POVL of 0.0235% for all operations.[11] The highest rates of POVL were found in cardiac (0.086%) and spinal fusion surgery (0.03%). By contrast, POVL after appendectomy was 0.0012% and after laminectomy without fusion was 0.0086%.[11] In a retrospective study using NIS data, Patil and colleagues found that the overall incidence of POVL after spine surgery was 0.094%, though they used slightly different years and inclusion and exclusion criteria for data analysis.[18] Estimates for ION after spine surgery were 0.017% from derived NIS data.[18]

OUTCOMES

Recovery of vision after POVL is difficult to assess accurately, as the vast majority of literature is retrospective and patients may have had no follow-up or have been examined at inconsistent times after the event. Additionally, though visual acuity may improve to normal or near normal in the unaffected portion of the visual field, significant scotoma or altitudinal field cuts may still exist. In Hollenhorst et al.'s first description of eight cases of CRAO associated with the horseshoe headrest in the prone position, they described full recovery of visual acuity in two of eight patients, though small residual blind spots or scotoma still lingered.[19] The third patient out of eight had good recovery of visual acuity (20/60) in the normal visual field but had a large residual central scotoma. An additional two patients had final visual acuity of hand motion only with small preserved isles of vision, and the remaining three patients had no recovery of vision and no light perception in the affected eye. In Roth's review of the literature of 32 cases of CRAO of more minor branch retinal artery occlusion (BRAO), 53% of patients had no recovery of vision, and 43% of cases had no information provided on recovery.[13] In the American Society of Anesthesiologists (ASA) POVL Registry, which collected cases of visual loss nationally, occurring after nonocular surgery, the authors found that only 2 of 10 patients with CRAO associated with prone spine surgery had any degree of recovery.[12]

Patients who develop cortical blindness frequently have good recovery of vision in contrast to patients who develop CRAO, AION, or PION. Recovery may depend on the severity and duration of insult and degree of collateral flow when hypoperfusion is the etiology. Two-thirds of patients reviewed by Roth reported some improvement in vision.[13]

Outcomes for AION and PION are similar to those for CRAO with poor recovery in most cases. Only 29% to 42% of patients with perioperative ION report any recovery, and none of the patients reported a return to baseline vision.[12,13,21] However, Ho and colleagues in their literature review of ION cases occurring after spine surgery found that 60% to 65% of patients had some improvement at follow-up.[22]

RISK FACTORS

Risk factors for POVL have been difficult to conduct because of the relatively low incidence of this complication. Some studies have been limited by use of multiple

POVL diagnoses in one group, lack of significant numbers of affected POVL patients, use of specific POVL diagnoses obtained from widely disparate operations, lack of verifiable information, and lack of detailed perioperative data, such as operative duration and blood loss.

RISK FACTORS FOR POVL AND ION

In 1997, Myers et al. published the first case–control study comparing 28 patients who developed POVL after spinal fusion surgery to patients who underwent similar spine operations who did not develop POVL.[23] They identified longer operative duration and larger blood loss as significant risk factors, whereas lowest hematocrit and lowest blood pressure did not differ between groups. This study was remarkable primarily because it demonstrated that POVL after spine surgery was becoming a significant perioperative complication nationally. Their findings of a lack of significance with respect to lowest hematocrit and lowest blood pressure, and visual loss stimulated interest in research to determine the predisposing risk factors in these cases. However, because they combined all POVL diagnoses including cortical blindness, CRAO, and all ION cases, whose etiologies are thought to differ, it is difficult to draw conclusions from their data.

Despite these methodological issues, Holy et al. in 2009 performed a retrospective cohort study at one institution examining risk factors specifically for perioperative ION and also found no significant differences in blood pressure or lowest hematocrit between 17 patients who developed ION and those who did not.[24] They were not able to identify any risk factors associated with ION, including co-existing conditions of higher body mass index (BMI), diabetes, smoking, hypertension, stroke history, coronary artery disease, myocardial infarction, renal disease, or hyperlipidemia. Further, they found no differences between groups on fundoscopic examination of a "disc-at-risk," signifying a small cup-to-disc ratio, and a putative risk factor for the development of spontaneous ION. Although these authors examined only cases of ION, they combined cases from widely disparate procedures including spine surgery, cardiac surgery, and others. If different procedures have different etiologies for causing ION, it is possible that this type of analysis may have missed risk factors unique to the development of ION in specific procedures such as the prone position.

In a retrospective analysis of 602 patients who underwent open heart surgery, the development of anterior ischemic optic neuropathy was associated with prolonged cardiopulmonary bypass times, low hematocrit levels,

excessive perioperative body weight gain, and the use of epinephrine and amrinone.[25] In a matched case–control study of ION after cardiopulmonary bypass, Nuttall et al. found that patients with clinically significant and severe vascular disease history, preoperative angiogram within 48 hours of surgery, and lower postoperative hemoglobin were at increased risk for ION.[26] They speculated that the risk factor for preoperative angiogram within 48 hours of surgery may have been related to more severe disease, more urgent nature of surgery, or the increased risk of red blood cell transfusion associated with angiograms just prior to surgery.

RISK FACTORS FOR POVL DERIVED FROM NIS DATABASE STUDIES

Two studies using the NIS database for examining risk factors for POVL were published in 2008 and 2009.[11,18] The study of Patil and colleagues[18] examined POVL cases associated with spine surgery between the years of 1993 and 2002. For non-ION, non-CRAO visual loss (primarily cortical blindness), the most significant risk factor reported was age <18 years (odds ratio [OR] 5.8, 95% confidence interval [CI] 4.33–7.80) and age >84 years (OR 3.2, 95% CI 2.07–5.08). They reported the following risk factors for ION associated with spine surgery after multivariate analysis: middle age (45- to 64-year-olds compared to 18- to 44-year-olds, OR 3.7, 95% CI 1.26–10.92); peripheral vascular disease (OR 6.4, 95% CI 2.18–18.55), diabetes (OR 2.3, 95% CI 1.06–4.79), anemia (OR 5.9, 95% CI 3.15–11.07), blood transfusion (OR 4.3, 95% CI 1.69–10.80), and hypotension (OR 10.1, 95% CI 2.85–35.84). As mentioned previously, the NIS database has poor reliability for determining risk factors associated with complications because of the inherent bias in assessment and data collection on patients with complications. Moreover, in this specific study, the findings of hypotension and anemia may be surrogate markers for prolonged surgery in the prone position, prolonged duration, blood loss, fluid administration, and other variables that are never collected in the NIS database but may have critical etiologic contributions to the development of ION. In fact, none of the "risk factors" identified in this study were found to be independent predictors of ION in the subsequent and largest case–control study performed to date to determine risk factors for ION and spine surgery.[27]

Shen et al.'s study using the NIS database for the years 1996–2005 was far more cautious in their data analysis by limiting the examined variables to data that were more consistently collected on all patients.[11] They found that after multivariable logistic regression, POVL incidence was significantly increased ($p < 0.001$) in patients undergoing nonfusion orthopedic surgery, spinal fusion surgery, and cardiac surgery compared to abdominal surgery patients (Table 11.2). Patients younger than 18 years had the highest risk for POVL in all procedures compared to 18- to 49-year-olds, primarily because of a higher risk for cortical blindness. Patients older than 50 years were at greater risk of developing ION and retinal vascular occlusion in all procedures. There was a significantly higher prevalence of POVL with male gender, Charlson comorbidity index >0, anemia, and blood transfusion.[11]

For ION in all procedures, Shen and colleagues found that age >50 was associated with a less than 2-fold increased risk in all procedures, as was male sex (Table 11.2).[11] Nonfusion orthopedic surgery, spinal fusion surgery, and cardiac surgery were all associated with a significantly increased risk of developing ION ($p < 0.001$).

For spine surgery in Shen's study, multivariable logistic regression demonstrated a greater than 4-fold increase in the risk of POVL for posterior spine surgery compared to anterior spine surgery ($p < 0.0001$, Table 11.2).[11] Children <18 years undergoing spine surgery had a more than 18-fold increase in the risk of POVL compared to 18- to 50-year-olds ($p < 0.0001$), primarily because of cortical blindness; and men were almost twice as likely ($p = 0.002$) as women to develop POVL after spine surgery (Table 11.2). Although the presence of anemia was identified as an independent risk factor after multivariate analysis ($p = 0.03$), confounding variables such as operative duration and blood loss were not available for analysis in the NIS database.

RISK FACTORS FOR ION AFTER SPINAL FUSION SURGERY USING A MULTICENTER CASE–CONTROL STUDY

At present, the most robust data available for identifying risk factors specifically for ION after spinal fusion surgery were obtained from the ASA POVL Registry.[12,27] The ASA POVL Registry was created in 1999 to collect cases of POVL occurring after nonocular surgery. A report of the perioperative profile of 93 POVL cases after spine surgery in 2006 indicated that 10 patients had experienced CRAO and 83 patients ION.[12] The patients with ION were noted to have 94% of cases with ≥6 hours anesthetic duration (a surrogate for operative duration) and 84% with ≥1000 ml estimated blood loss. Notably, 72% of the patients were men. Although this perioperative profile was useful, identification of risk factors required comparison of these ION cases to patients who underwent similar procedures but did not develop ION.

Subsequently, the ION cases associated with prone spinal fusion surgery from the ASA POVL Registry were used in a multicenter case–control study to determine risk factors for this complication.[27] Seventeen centers from across North America that performed a large volume of spinal fusion operations contributed controls for this study that were matched by year of surgery to minimize changes in practice patterns over time. Four controls for each ION case were randomly selected from a database of over 43,000 control spinal fusion operations. Inclusion criteria for cases and controls were 1) age ≥18 years; 2) a spinal fusion operation that was the first or only spine surgery on index admission and in which at least a portion of the procedure was in the prone position; 3) spinal surgery including the thoracic, lumbar, or sacral segments; 4) occurrence between 1991 and 2006; and 5) anesthetic duration of ≥4 hours. Cases and controls were excluded for incomplete medical records and any history of perioperative stroke or cardiopulmonary resuscitation on index admission. Cases were excluded for multiple staged procedures on index admission preceding onset of ION. Controls were excluded for any new onset of POVL on index admission. In the final analysis after controls were randomized and inclusion and exclusion criteria were met, a total of 80 ION cases were matched to 315 control cases.[27]

In the univariate analysis, investigators found that a significantly ($p < 0.05$) higher proportion of ION cases were associated with male sex, obesity, diabetes, use of the Wilson frame, longer anesthetic duration, greater blood loss, lowest intraoperative hematocrit, blood pressure >40% below baseline for 30 minutes, increased total volume replacement, increased total nonblood replacement, and lower percent colloid in the nonblood replacement.[27] Multivariate stepwise logistic regression identified six significant ($p < 0.05$) and independent risk factors for developing ION after spinal fusion surgery: male sex, obesity, use of Wilson frame, longer anesthetic duration, greater estimated blood loss, and decreased percent colloid administration (Table 11.3).

With the exception of male sex, the risk factors identified in this study are consistent with, but do not prove, the theory that venous congestion in the prone position for prolonged duration may predispose to the development of interstitial edema from capillary leak, decreased venous outflow, and decreased optic nerve perfusion.[27] Obese abdomens in the prone position lead to greater increases in central venous pressure; Wilson frames place the head much lower than the heart level; increased duration and blood loss lend to greater fluid shifts, inflammation, and edema formation as well as provide additional time for this injury to develop; and lower-percent

Table 11.2 RISK FACTORS FOR POSTOPERATIVE VISUAL LOSS (POVL)*

ALL PROCEDURES		ODDS RATIO	95% CONFIDENCE INTERVAL	*P* VALUE
Risk of any POVL	**Surgery Type**			
	Abdominal surgery	Referent		<0.001
	Nonfusion orthopedic	2.03	1.53–2.69	
	Spinal fusion	5.55	3.81–8.09	
	Cardiac	11.1	8.35–14.7	
	Age (years)			
	<18	6.91	4.3–11.1	<0.001
	18–49	Referent		
	50–64	1.51	1.18–1.94	
	≥65	1.99	1.55–2.56	
	Male	1.32	1.16–15.0	<0.001
	Charlson index ≥2 (referent0)	1.95	1.53–2.50	<0.001
Risk of ION	**Surgery Type**			
	Abdominal	Referent		
	Nonfusion orthopedic	1.89	1.09–3.27	<0.001
	Spinal fusion	6.96	3.8–12.8	
	Cardiac	8.04	4.57–14.2	
	Age (years)			
	<50	Referent		
	50–64	1.75	1.13–2.71	0.04
	≥65	1.65	1.05–2.60	
	Male	2.04	1.47–2.82	<0.001
SPINAL FUSION SURGERY		**ODDS RATIO**	**95% CONFIDENCE INTERVAL**	*P* VALUE
Risk of any POVL	**Position**			
	Anterior	Referent		
	Posterior	4.16	2.13–8.13	<0.001
	Other	2.69	1.09–6.62	
	Age (years)			
	<18	18.3	9.81–34.0	<0.001
	18–49	Referent		
	50–64	1.65	0.90–3.03	
	≥65	2.07	1.12–3.80	
	Male	1.75	1.22–2.50	0.002

*Modified from Shen Y et al. The prevalence of perioperative visual loss in the United States: A 10-year study from 1996 to 2005 of spinal, orthopedic, cardiac, and general surgery. *Anesth Analg* 2009;109:1534–1545. Data from the Nationwide Inpatient Sample. Only risk factors with OR ≥1.3 after multivariable analysis are displayed in Table 11.2. ION, ischemic optic neuropathy.

colloid may lead to greater edema formation in the short term of an operation. The finding of male sex as an independent risk factor is consistent with NIS data, but its contribution to ION is unclear. The anatomy and blood supply of the eye and anterior visual pathways in men and women are not significantly different. There is a higher prevalence of Leber's hereditary optic neuropathy in males, and Giordano et al. showed a therapeutic benefit for estrogen-like molecules in Leber's optic neuropathy.[28] This may indicate that estrogen has some protective effect on the optic nerve.

The Postoperative Visual Loss Study Group found no statistically significant independent effect on ION of older age,

Table 11.3 RISK FACTORS FOR ISCHEMIC OPTIC
NEUROPATHY AFTER SPINAL FUSION SURGERY
(THE POVL STUDY GROUP, *ANESTHESIOLOGY*, 2012)*

	ODDS RATIO	95% CONFIDENCE INTERVAL	*P* VALUE
Male	2.53	1.35–4.91	0.005
Obesity	2.83	1.52–5.39	0.001
Use of Wilson frame	4.30	2.13–8.75	<0.001
Estimated blood loss, OR per liter	1.39	1.22–1.58	<0.001
Anesthetic duration, OR per hour	1.34	1.13–1.61	<0.001
% Colloid in nonblood volume	0.67	0.52–0.82	<0.001

Modified from The Postoperative Visual Loss Study Group. Risk factors associated with ischemic optic neuropathy after spinal fusion surgery. *Anesthesiology* 2012;116:15–24. Risk factors identified after multivariate regression analysis from a multicenter case–control study comparing 80 cases of ischemic optic neuropathy after spinal fusion surgery to 315 controls undergoing similar spinal fusion surgery and matched by year of surgery.

hypertension, atherosclerosis, smoking, or diabetes in patients undergoing spinal fusion, and they suggested that the etiology of ION may be more strongly influenced by intraoperative physiologic perturbations than by any known pre-existing disease or vasculopathy.[27] Almost as important as what this study found as independent risk factors for ION after spinal fusion surgery are the multiple purported risk factors from case reports and case series that were not found to be significant and independent risk factors for ION. The collection in this study of intraoperative variables such as blood loss, anesthetic duration, fluid administration, and type of surgical frame demonstrated that the frequently suggested risk factors of hypotension and anemia were possibly surrogate markers for these very prolonged operations in the prone position with large blood loss. It highlights the limitations of the NIS database for determining risk factors for complications associated with intraoperative events. Additionally, by the time this study was devised, sufficient evidence existed that predisposing variables for ION between cardiac bypass procedures and prone spine surgery procedures might differ, thus highlighting the need to compare cases with similar types of ophthalmologic injury (e.g., ION) from similar types of surgical procedures to controls from similar types of surgical procedures.

As always, data from retrospective case–control studies must be regarded with caution. Significant limitations exist with respect to collection of data from the cases and controls, including selection bias, lack of standardized methodology for measuring and recording blood pressure and hematocrit values, the effect of coincidental occurrence of variables, table tilt, and others. Moreover, cases were collected from a different mix of institutions than that for the controls. Further, it is possible that variables excluded in the multivariate logistic regression, but significant in the univariate analsysis, had a significant contributory effect on the development of ION.[27] Practitioners are advised to use sound clinical judgement when caring for these complex spinal fusion patients, and to avoid extreme physiologic perturbations when possible.

PREVENTIVE STRATEGIES AND TREATMENT FOR ION

PREVENTIVE STRATEGIES FOR ION

Because ION is a relatively uncommon complication, randomized, controlled studies evaluating the effect of an intervention on the development of ION have not been performed. Furthermore, they are not likely to be conducted in the near future because of the ethical concerns and enormous cost and number of centers over many years that would be required to adequately power a study of this nature. Consequently, untested preventive strategies for ION include minimizing the effect of independent risk factors identified in the largest case–control study to date with detailed perioperative data.[27] Changing male sex and BMI are not rational or likely areas to modify risk, but patient selection and degree of surgical invasiveness when pre-existing risk factors are present can potentially influence the incidence of ION. Selection of surgical frames that keep the head neutral with the heart, and positioning the surgical table so that the head is neutral or higher than the heart may help minimize venous congestion in the head. Perfomance of surgeries by skilled, experienced surgeons can minimize duration and blood loss in the prone position. Further, modification of fluid administration such that colloids are used along with crystalloids may also decrease the occurrence of ION.

However, models of risk are based on statistics for a given set of patients and do not necessarily equate to models of prevention for all populations. Unidentified risk factors may still place patients at elevated risk for ION, as well as the seemingly multifactorial nature of this injury. Stevens et al. reported three cases[17] of ION after major spinal fusion surgery in two women and one man where the percent of colloid (5% albumin) in the nonblood volume administered was 13.6%, 25.9%, and 37%, far above the average 8% colloid found in the control group in the large multicenter case–control study.[27] Yet, these three cases all had an operative duration of 6 or more hours, blood loss ranging from 875 ml to 9000 ml, unknown BMI, and use of unknown surgical frames, thereby increasing risk from other contributory factors. Although research on this complication is difficult because of the low incidence, we must continue to evaluate our incidence of ION after spinal fusion surgery, retest statistical models for predicting ION, and evaluate the effect of any interventions, if even on a historical basis.

TREATMENT FOR ION

There are various treatment methods that have been attempted but not rigorously studied because of the same inherent limitations in identifying risk factors for low-incidence complications. Perhaps the three most common interventions noted in the literature include elevation of blood pressure to normal or supranormal values, transfusion of red blood cells to hematocrit values over 30%, and use of high-dose systemic corticosteroids.[17,22] Results have been varied, ranging from no improvement to significant improvement in vision. Elevation of the head is a relatively benign intervention that may improve periorbital edema and venous congestion quickly, but it may also result in hypovolemic hypotension. It may occasionally conflict with the surgeon's desire to leave the patient supine if there is a concurrent dural tear. Use of diphenylhydantoin, acetazolamide, mannitol, and hyperbaric oxygen therapy have also been suggested but lack proven benefit. A careful risk–benefit assessment should be made when using unproven therapies because of significant risks associated with vasopressor use and transfusion, infection risk with steroids, hypovolemia with mannitol, and transportation issues associated with delivering hyperbaric oxygen in the acute postoperative setting.

CURRENT GUIDELINES AND RECOMMENDATIONS

The following recommendations for patients undergoing major spinal surgery in the prone position are based on the recently updated ASA Task Force on Perioperative Blindness.[29]

The Task Force believes that there may be an increased risk of ION in patients who undergo prolonged procedures, have substantial blood loss, or both. These patients are referred to as "high-risk patients."

1. Consider informing patients in whom prolonged spine surgery, substantial blood loss, or both are anticipated, that there is a small unpredictable risk of POVL.

2. Continually monitor the blood pressure and consider use of central venous pressure monitoring in high-risk patients.

3. Colloids should be used along with crystalloids to maintain intravascular volume in patients who have substantial blood loss.

4. Hemoglobin or hematocrit should be monitored periodically during surgery in patients who experience substantial blood loss.

5. Position the head at or above the level of heart. The head should be maintained in a neutral forward position (e.g., without significant neck flexion, extension, lateral flexion, or rotation) when possible.

6. Avoid direct pressure on the globe, to prevent CRAO.

7. Consider staging spine procedures in high-risk patients.

8. A high-risk patient's vision should be assessed when a patient becomes alert.

9. If there is concern for POVL, an urgent ophthalmologic consultation should be obtained.

10. Additional management may include optimizing hemoglobin/hematocrit values, hemodynamic status, and arterial oxygenation.

11. Consider magnetic resonance imaging to rule out intracranial causes of POVL.

12. The Task Force could not find a role for antiplatelet agents, steroids, or intraocular pressure-lowering agents in the treatment of perioperative ION.

The Task Force did not find an association of POVL with deliberate hypotension, a documented lower limit of hemoglobin concentration, or use of vasopressors; therefore, the use of deliberate hypotension, a transfusion threshold, and use of vasopressors should be determined on a case-by-case basis.

CONCLUSIONS

POVL is an uncommon but potentially devastating complication associated primarily with cardiac bypass procedures, major spine surgery, and head and neck operations; it can also present after a wide variety of miscellaneous cases. The major types of POVL include CRAO, cortical blindness, AION, and PION. CRAO is most often associated with spine surgery in the prone position from globe compression that can be easily prevented by frequent eye checks. Emboli less commonly cause perioperative CRAO. Recovery from CRAO is poor and there is no known treatment. Perioperative cortical blindness is typically associated with procedures with high embolic loads or profound hypoperfusion with watershed infarctions of the cerebral cortex. Recovery from cortical blindness is frequently good in approximately two-thirds of cases.

Perioperative ION is increased in cardiac bypass procedures, spinal fusion surgery, and nonfusion orthopedic surgery. It is most often observed after cardiac bypass procedures where AION predominates. Risk factors for ION in this setting have been reported as prolonged cardiopulmonary bypass times, low hematocrit levels, excessive perioperative body weight gain, the use of epinephrine and amrinone, clinically significant and severe vascular disease, preoperative angiogram within 48 hours of surgery, and low postoperative hemoglobin. Perioperative ION after prone spine surgery is more frequently PION. Significant and independent risk factors for ION after prone spine surgery include male gender, obesity, use of the Wilson frame, prolonged operative duration, increased blood loss, and lower percent colloid in the nonblood volume administration.

Treatment for perioperative ION, regardless of etiology, has not been proven but is most frequently aimed at correcting significant hypotension and/or anemia. Recovery from perioperative ION is poor in most series, with improvement in less than half of patients and vision almost never returning to baseline. The ASA Task Force on Perioperative Visual Loss recently updated the advisory for the prevention of perioperative blindness after spine surgery, which provides some guidance on the management of these complex cases.

CONFLICT OF INTEREST STATEMENT

V.K.R. and L.A.L have no conflicts of interest to disclose.

REFERENCES

1. Lee LA, Newman NJ, Wagner TA, Dettori JR, Dettori NJ. Postoperative ischemic optic neuropathy. *Spine.* 2010;35(9 Suppl):S105–S116.
2. Appelt GL, Benson GS, Corriere JN, Jr. Transient blindness: unusual initial symptom of transurethral prostatic resection reaction. *Urology.* 1979;13(4):402–404.
3. Gartner S, Billet E. Acute glaucoma: as a complication of general surgery. *Am J Ophthalmol.* 1958;45(5):668–671.
4. Vote BJ, Hart RH, Worsley DR, Borthwick JH, Laurent S, McGeorge AJ. Visual loss after use of nitrous oxide gas with general anesthetic in patients with intraocular gas still persistent up to 30 days after vitrectomy. *Anesthesiology.* 2002;97(5):1305–1308.
5. Roth S. Perioperative visual loss: what do we know, what can we do? *Br J Anaesth* 2009; 103(suppl 1):i31–i40.
6. Yi JH, Ha SH, Kim YK, Choi EM. Posterior reversible encephalopathy syndrome in an untreated hypertensive patient after spinal surgery under general anesthesia—a case report. *Korean J Anesthesiol.* 2011;60(5):369–372.
7. Levin LA. Optic nerve. In: Kaufman PL, Alm A, Adler FH, eds. *Adler's Physiology of the Eye.* 10th ed. St. Louis, MO: Mosby; 2003: 603–638.
8. Cioffi GA, Granstam E, Alm A. Ocular circulation. In: Kaufman PL, Alm A, Adler FH, eds. *Adler's Physiology of the Eye.* 10th ed. St. Louis: Mosby; 2003:747–784.
9. Pillunat LE, Anderson DR, Knighton RW, Joos KM, Feuer WJ. Autoregulation of human optic nerve head circulation in response to increased intraocular pressure. *Exp Eye Res.* 1997;64(5):737–744.
10. Blunt MJ, Steele EJ. The blood supply of the optic nerve and chiasma in man. *J Anat.* 1956;90(4):486–493.
11. Shen Y, Drum M, Roth S. The prevalence of perioperative visual loss in the United States: a 10-year study from 1996 to 2005 of spinal, orthopedic, cardiac, and general surgery. *Anesth Analg.* 2009;109(5): 1534–1545.
12. Lee LA, Roth S, Posner KL, et al. The American Society of Anesthesiologists Postoperative Visual Loss Registry: analysis of 93 spine surgery cases with postoperative visual loss. *Anesthesiology.* 2006;105(4):652–659.
13. Roth S. Postoperative Visual loss. In: Miller RD, Eriksson LI, Fleisher LA, Wiener-Kronish JP, Young WL, eds. *Miller's Anesthesia.* Vol 2. 7th ed. Philadelphia: Churchill Livingstone/Elsevier; 2009:2821–2841.
14. Warner ME, Warner MA, Garrity JA, MacKenzie RA, Warner DO. The frequency of perioperative vision loss. *Anesth Analg.* 2001;93(6):1417–1421, table of contents.
15. Roth S, Barach P. Postoperative visual loss: still no answers—yet. *Anesthesiology.* 2001;95(3):575–577.
16. Chang SH, Miller NR. The incidence of vision loss due to perioperative ischemic optic neuropathy associated with spine surgery: the Johns Hopkins Hospital Experience. *Spine.* 2005;30(11):1299–1302.
17. Stevens WR, Glazer PA, Kelley SD, Lietman TM, Bradford DS. Ophthalmic complications after spinal surgery. *Spine* 1997;22(12): 1319–1324.
18. Patil CG, Lad EM, Lad SP, Ho C, Boakye M. Visual loss after spine surgery: a population-based study. *Spine.* 2008;33(13): 1491–1496.
19. Hollenhorst RW, Svien HJ, Benoit CF. Unilateral blindness occurring during anesthesia for neurosurgical operations. *AMA Arch Ophthalmol.* 1954;52(6):819–830.
20. Roth S, Gillesberg I. Injuries to the visual system and other sense organs. In: Benumof J, Saidman LJ, eds. *Anesthesia & Perioperative Complications.* 2nd ed. St Louis: Mosby; 1999:377–408.
21. Sadda SR, Nee M, Miller NR, Biousse V, Newman NJ, Kouzis A. Clinical spectrum of posterior ischemic optic neuropathy. *Am J Ophthalmol.* 2001;132(5):743–750.
22. Ho VT, Newman NJ, Song S, Ksiazek S, Roth S. Ischemic optic neuropathy following spine surgery. *J Neurosurg Anesthesiol.* 2005;17(1):38–44.
23. Myers MA, Hamilton SR, Bogosian AJ, Smith CH, Wagner TA. Visual loss as a complication of spine surgery. A review of 37 cases. *Spine.* 1997;22(12):1325–1329.

24. Holy SE, Tsai JH, McAllister RK, Smith KH. Perioperative ischemic optic neuropathy: a case control analysis of 126,666 surgical procedures at a single institution. *Anesthesiology*. 2009;110(2):246–253.

25. Shapira OM, Kimmel WA, Lindsey PS, Shahian DM. Anterior ischemic optic neuropathy after open heart operations. *Ann Thorac Surg*.1996;61(2):660–666.

26. Nuttall GA, Garrity JA, Dearani JA, Abel MD, Schroeder DR, Mullany CJ. Risk factors for ischemic optic neuropathy after cardiopulmonary bypass: a matched case/control study. *Anesth Analg*. 2001;93(6):1410–1416, table of contents.

27. The Postoperative Visual Loss Study Group. Risk factors associated with ischemic optic neuropathy after spinal fusion surgery. *Anesthesiology*. 2012;116(1):15–24.

28. Giordano C, Montopoli M, Perli E, et al. Oestrogens ameliorate mitochondrial dysfunction in Leber's hereditary optic neuropathy. *Brain* 2011;134(Pt 1):220–234.

29. Practice advisory for perioperative visual loss associated with spine surgery: an updated report by the American Society of Anesthesiologists Task Force on Perioperative Visual Loss. *Anesthesiology*. 2012;116(2):274–285.

PART IV

FUTURE DIRECTIONS

12.

STANDARDS FOR INTRAOPERATIVE NEUROPHYSIOLOGIC MONITORING

Antoun Koht, J. Richard Toleikis, and Tod B. Sloan

INTRODUCTION

As discussed elsewhere in this volume, surgery on or near the central nervous system carries risks of neurologic compromise either from the pathology that prompted the surgery or as a consequence of the procedure itself. Currently, electroencephalography (EEG), electromyography (EMG), somatosensory evoked potentials (SSEPs), auditory brainstem responses (ABRs), and motor evoked potentials (MEPs) are the most commonly employed electrophysiological monitoring techniques for assessing and protecting neurologic function during surgery. Their use has become the standard for improving surgical decision making and reducing neurologic complications.[1-13]

Use of these techniques is based on acquiring and measuring the activity from the various neural pathways that mediate the activity or responses. Since these responses often correlate with clinical function, monitoring provides a means for assessing the functional status of the nervous system. This differs from the use of traditional physiological monitors (e.g., blood pressure and oxygenation), which only measure parameters that are supportive of function. Although not a replacement for the awake neurologic exam, intraoperative neurophysiologic monitoring provides a means for detecting electrophysiological changes that result from unfavorable surgical or physiological events and in so doing prompt the initiation of surgical or physiological maneuvers that can reverse the damaging events and reduce postoperative morbidity. A discussion of each of these techniques and their current and future application follows.

ELECTROPHYSIOLOGICAL MONITORING METHODS

ELECTROENCEPHALOGRAPHY (EEG)

EEG represents the summated synaptic activity of the pyramidal cells of the superficial layers of the cerebral cortex. This synaptic activity represents approximately 40–50% of the resting metabolic activity of the cortical neurons and reflects the interneuronal communication and "pacemaker" centers that drive rhythmic synaptic firing. Since the amplitude of the synaptic potentials is small, the activity recorded in electrodes on the scalp represents a small volume of cortical activity beneath the electrode (2–3 cm in diameter). As such, EEG recordings are usually done with a large number of electrodes to cover the cortical surface, or a smaller number strategically placed near regions where the procedure places that brain region at risk. Although EEG is affected by anesthetic agents, once a baseline rhythm is established, monitoring can detect global or focal abnormalities that warn of neuronal compromise.

Three major applications of EEG are based on its response to changes in metabolic activity. One of its widest applications is a result of EEG being particularly sensitive to ischemia, making it useful during surgery in which the risk of stroke from reduced blood flow to the brain can occur. When cerebral blood flow is reduced from normal (50 cc/min/100 g) the electrical activity becomes altered (at about 20–22 cc/min/100 g) and eventually lost (at about 15 cc/min/100 g). With complete cessation of blood flow, EEG responds rapidly with a total loss of activity within 20–30 seconds. Fortunately, neuronal infarction does not occur immediately; neuronal death occurs after 3–4 hours of ischemia at 16–17 cc/min/100 g, and at progressively shorter time periods as the blood flow is reduced further (Figure 12.1).[14]

The goal of monitoring is to identify an ischemic condition as soon as possible to encourage maneuvers in order to increase blood flow or reduce the time of the ischemia and to reduce the potential for neural injury. For example, when an ischemic condition occurs, blood pressure may be increased to improve the neural environment and potentially improve outcomes. Monitoring can also be used to determine if the maneuvers used to improve unfavorable neurologic circumstances are effective. This has made the use of EEG monitoring valuable during procedures such as carotid endarterectomies and intracranial vascular surgeries (for aneurysms and arteriovenous [AV] malformations).

A second use for EEG during surgery is to monitor cerebral metabolic activity when intentional depression of metabolism is used to improve the energy supply–demand balance, thus increasing the tolerance to ischemia. This reduction in metabolism can be accomplished using drugs such as barbiturates, which can stop synaptic activity (thus reducing

metabolism to 40–50% of normal), or by using hypothermia, which can reduce all metabolic activity (basal and synaptic). As a result, EEG monitoring is used during procedures to verify suppression and to guide the degree of pharmacologic suppression; burst suppression is usually used as an endpoint since it represents near maximal suppression.

A third use for EEG is to identify seizure activity. In the operating room, this can be used during operations in which seizures are a consequence of cortical stimulation, such as those used to identify the motor cortex or the eloquent regions for speech (e.g., Broca's or Wernicke's area). This can be done in conjunction with surgery in which identification of a native seizure area is to be accomplished for the purpose of resection, while minimizing damage to the eloquent cortical regions.[15] Monitoring for seizure activity can also be used in the intensive care unit (ICU) to identify otherwise undetected seizure activity and to guide patient management when the associated hypermetabolism produces an unfavorable relative ischemia.

ELECTROMYOGRAPHY (EMG)

Similar to monitoring the spontaneous activity of EEG, recording the spontaneous activity of muscles (EMG) can be used to identify irritation or stimulation of nerve roots and peripheral or cranial nerves. Under anesthesia, this muscle activity is usually quiescent so that when the nerve is stimulated or irritated, the resulting muscle activity signals that event. In addition to observing unintentional irritation of the nerve, electrical stimulation can be used to identify the nerve or assess its integrity. As with the other responses, the EMG activity can be observed as a display of electrical activity over time or can be played over a loud speaker to give direct feedback to the surgeon.

Two types of nonstimulated responses can often be seen during monitoring (Figure 12.2):[16] brief discharges, caused by mechanical or metabolic stimuli, and high-frequency intermittent or continuous bursts. Causes of irritation include mechanical stimulation (e.g., nearby dissection; ultrasonic aspiration or drilling), nerve retraction, thermal irritation (e.g., heating from irrigation, lasers, drilling, or electrocautery), and chemical or metabolic insults.[2] Long trains of activity should raise concerns because they are associated with impending nerve injury (nerve compression, traction, or other injurious forces, such as heating from nearby drilling).[3] Their audible sounds have been likened to the sound of an outboard motor boat engine, swarming bees, "popcorn" popping, or an aircraft engine ("bomber") potentials.

Cranial nerve monitoring is of particular interest as cranial nerves are susceptible to damage intraoperatively because

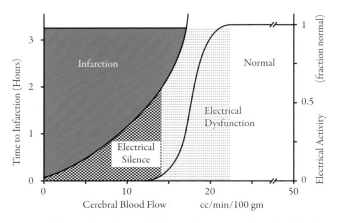

Figure 12.1 Relationship of cortical electrical activity and cerebral blood flow and infarction. Depiction of electrical activity and the occurrence of irreversible cell death (infarction) as cerebral blood flow is reduced from normal (50 cc/min/100 g). As shown here, the EEG becomes abnormal below 22 cc/min/100 g and persistently suppressed when blood flow reaches 15 cc/min/100 g. Infarction occurs at 17–18 cc/min/100 g after 3–4 hours and after progressively shorter periods when blood flow is below this level Reproduced from Sloan and Jameson (2012)[14] with permission.

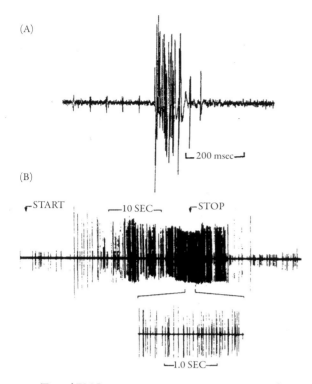

(A)

⌐ 200 msec ⌐

(B)

⌐START   ⌐10 SEC⌐   ⌐STOP

⌐1.0 SEC⌐

Figure 12.2 Typical EMG responses seen in surgery; EMG recordings from muscle during surgery near motor nerves. The upper trace (**A**) shows a single, brief burst of muscle activity from nerve irritation. The lower trace (**B**) shows sustained "neurotonic" activity from injurious nerve irritation. Note the difference in time scales   Reproduced from Prass et al. (1987)16 with permission.

Table 12.1 CRANIAL NERVE MONITORING

CRANIAL NERVE	MUSCLES MONITORED
III	Oculomotor: Inferior rectus m.
IV	Trochlear: superior oblique m.
V	Trigeminal: masseter m. and/or temporalis m.
VI	Abducens: lateral rectus m.
VII	Facial: orbicularis oculi m. and/or orbicularis oris m.
IX	Glossopharyngeal: stylopharyngeus m. (posterior soft palate)
X	Vagus: vocal folds, cricothyroid m.
XI	Spinal accessory: sternocleidomastoid m. and/or trapezius m.
XII	Hypoglossal: genioglossus m. (tongue)

of their small sizes, limited epineurium, and complicated courses, which may be distorted by pathology. In addition, they may be intertwined in a tumor destined for resection. The damage to these nerves occurs from trauma (surgical disruption, manipulation), and this leads to paresis or paralysis (with subsequent disability or deformity) and possibly pain.

Monitoring can be carried out by observation of the spontaneous activity of muscles (EMG) innervated by the relevant cranial nerve, or by response to stimulation, which can be used to locate the nerve in the operative field or to confirm nerve integrity. All cranial nerves with a motor component can be monitored by means of their respectively innervated muscles (Table 12.1). For peripheral nerves and nerve roots, typical muscles used for monitoring purposes are shown Table 12.2.

SOMATOSENSORY EVOKED POTENTIALS (SSEPS)

One of the most commonly acquired responses used for monitoring purposes is the somatosensory evoked potential (SSEP).[9,17] This response is acquired by stimulating large, mixed nerves containing both motor and sensory components.

Typically, these responses are elicited by median, ulnar, or posterior tibial nerve stimulation. The stimulation activates both the motor and sensory components of the nerve. Activation of the motor components typically results in muscle twitches from distal musculature, whereas activation of the sensory components results in responses that ascend the sensory pathways to the brain. These cephalad traveling responses follow the pathways that mediate the sensations of proprioception and vibration. The responses enter the spinal cord via the posterior nerve roots and ascend in the ipsilateral dorsal column. The first synapses in these pathways occur near the nucleus cuneatus (for the upper extremities) and the nucleus

Table 12.2 MUSCLES TYPICALLY MONITORED FOR NERVE ROOT AND PERIPHERAL NERVE MONITORING

C 2–4	Trapezius, sternocleidomastoid
C 5, 6	Biceps, deltoid
C 6, 7	Flexor carpi radialis
C 8–T 1	Adductor pollicis brevis, abductor digiti minimi
T 5–6	Upper rectus abdominis
T 7–8	Middle rectus abdominis
T 9–11	Lower rectus abdominis
T 12	Inferior rectus abdominis
L 2	Adductor longus
L 2–4	Vastus medialis
L 4–S 1	Tibialis anterior
L 5–S 1	Peroneus longus
S1–2	Gastrocnemius
S 2–4	Anal sphincter

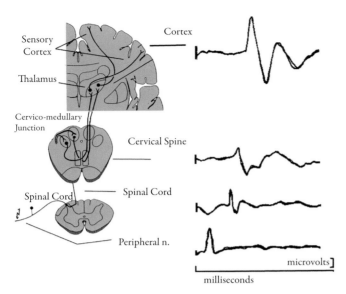

Figure 12.3 Pathway of the somatosensory evoked potential (SSEP). The SSEP is produced by stimulation of a peripheral nerve (arrow). The electrical activity enters via the dorsal nerve root and ascends the spinal cord via the dorsal column pathway, which transmits the senses of proprioception and vibration. It synapses at the cervicomedullary junction and crosses the midline, ascending in the medial lemniscus to the ventromedial nucleus of the thalamus where it has a second synapse. From there it ascends to the sensory cerebral cortex. SSEP recordings can be made along the pathway; responses from the peripheral nerve, spinal cord, cervical spine, and cerebral cortex are shown Reproduced from Jameson and Sloan (2006)89 with permission.

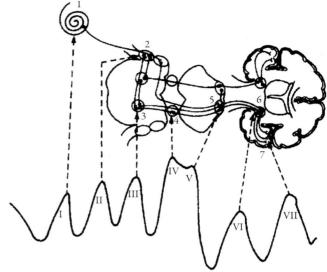

Figure 12.4 Pathway and peaks of the auditory brainstem response (ABR). The first seven peaks of the ABR are produced near the structures in the brainstem as described in the text. Typically waves I, III, and V are seen during monitoring Reproduced from Aravabhumi et al. (1987)18 with permission.

gracilis (for the lower extremities). The responses then cross the midline near the cervicomedullary junction and ascend through the brainstem via the contralateral medial lemniscus. A second synapse occurs in the ventroposterolateral nucleus of the thalamus. From there, the responses continue and ascend to the contralateral sensory cortex (Figure 12.3). The most commonly recorded responses are those recorded over the sensory cortex. However, the responses can also be recorded at other points along the pathway, including over peripheral nerves and the spinal cord.[17] These responses can be used to assess the functionality of those neural tissues that mediate the sensory responses, including the specific peripheral nerves, the spinal cord tracts, the brainstem pathways, and the cerebral cortex destinations.

AUDITORY BRAINSTEM RESPONSES (ABRS)

Another commonly used sensory evoked potential is the auditory brainstem response (ABR), which is produced when sound activates the cochlea and the electrical response is then conveyed by the neural pathways for hearing. The term *ABR* refers to the responses recorded from the brainstem, usually in the first 10 milliseconds after stimulation. This type of evoked potential has also been referred to as the brainstem auditory evoked response

(BAER) or brainstem auditory evoked potential (BAEP). After activating the cochlea, the resulting nerve impulses travel to the brainstem via the eighth cranial nerve. The nerve impulses then travel via the brainstem acoustic relay nuclei and lemniscal pathways to activate neurons in the auditory cortex. Three major peaks are usually seen in the monitored responses: waves I, III, and V[9,18] (Figure 12.4). Wave I is produced in the extracranial portion of CN VIII, wave III in the acoustic relay nuclei and tracts deep in the midline of the lower pons, and wave V in the lateral lemniscus and inferior colliculus of the contralateral pons. Occasionally, waves II and IV are also present. Responses to auditory stimulation can also be recorded over the sensory cortex and are termed middle latency auditory evoked responses.

As with the SSEP, the ABR is used to assess the neural pathway that produces and mediates the response. This includes the cochlea, the eighth cranial nerve, and the brainstem structures through which CN VIII traverses. The ABR waveforms are thought to be more sensitive to functional changes resulting from brainstem injuries than vital-sign abnormalities.[19]

DERMATOMAL AND VISUAL EVOKED RESPONSES

Sensory responses can also be acquired from stimulation of specific dermatomes of the body surface (dermatomal evoked potentials [DEPs]) or by stimulation of the eye by light flashes (visual evoked potentials [VEPs]). However, these reponses are rarely used for monitoring purposes because the VEP responses acquired during surgery have little correlation to the presence or loss of vision, and both the DEP and VEP responses are markedly affected by anesthesia, making them challenging to record.

MOTOR EVOKED POTENTIALS (MEPS)

Motor evoked potential (MEP) monitoring is one of the more recent additions to the electrophysiological monitoring armamentarium. A variety of methods have been used in the past to assess the functional status of the motor pathways, but it appears that they were not specific for monitoring the corticospinal tract. In particular, these methods employed stimulation of the spinal cord using epidural electrodes or electrodes placed near the spinal cord to elicit neurogenic responses from peripheral nerves in the lower extremities (e.g., so-called neurogenic motor evoked potentials [NMEPs]). However, this technique primarily activated sensory rather than motor pathways and has been abandoned as a technique for monitoring motor pathway function. The current MEP methods use stimulation of the motor cortex and have been adopted for monitoring corticospinal tract function.

Transcranial stimulation directly stimulates the pyramidal cells of the motor cortex, resulting in a wave of descending depolarization that involves 4–5% of the corticospinal tract (Figure 12.5).[12] When this wave of depolarization is recorded by electrodes in the epidural space, it is termed the "D" (direct) wave. Additional transsynaptic activation of internuncial pathways in the cortex results in a series of smaller waves called "I" (indirect) waves that follow the D wave. The motor pathway begins in the motor cortex and descends, crossing the midline in the lower lateral brainstem. It further descends in the ipsilateral and anterior funiculi of the spinal cord. The electrical activities of the D and I waves summate in the anterior horn cell, resulting in activation of peripheral nerves, which produce compound muscle action potentials (CMAPs) and visible body movements if a patient is not pharmacologically paralyzed or deeply anesthetized (e.g., with volatile anesthetic agents). Methods have been developed for stimulation of the motor cortex using brief, intense magnetic fields or electrical stimulation using a series of electrical pulses. Because of their sensitivity to anesthesia and the physical bulk of the magnetic stimulator, the magnetic technique has been supplanted by the electrical technique. Electrical stimulation can be applied to the scalp or directly to the brain (direct cortical stimulation [DCS]) when more focal stimulation and less body movements are desired.

Monitoring can be done by recording in the epidural space (D wave) and from muscles (CMAPs). The disadvantage of

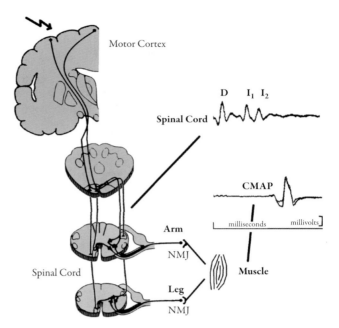

Figure 12.5 Pathway and typical responses of the motor evoked potential (MEP). MEPs are produced by stimulation of the motor cortex (arrow). The electrical activity descends following the corticospinal tract to the anterior horn of the spinal cord. After synapsing, the response then further descends to the peripheral nerve, traverses the neuromuscular junction, and produces a muscle response. The MEP can be measured in the epidural space as D and I waves, or as a compound muscle action potential (CMAP) Reproduced from Jameson (2006)12 with permission.

epidural recordings is that they do not differentiate laterality and require percutaneous or direct placement of the recording electrodes on the spine. However, the amplitudes of the D waves recorded in this manner are usually stable, and their amplitudes correlate with the number of functioning fibers of the corticospinal tract. Muscle recordings, in contrast, can differentiate unilateral changes and can be used to assess the functionality of specific nerves.

REFLEX RESPONSES

One other monitoring technique that is not widely used involves reflex responses. Examples of these reflex responses include blink reflexes, which involve the activation of cranial nerves, and those reflex responses resulting from stimulation of the pudendal nerve. The most common of these reflex response techniques is the H-reflex response, which is used to monitor spinal cord function.[6]

The H-reflex response is a CMAP recorded from muscle that results from electrical activation of a monosynaptic spinal cord reflex. The H reflex can be monitored following electrical stimulation of a peripheral nerve, which produces an initial motor response (M wave) and a simultaneous centrally traveling volley of activity in the sensory and motor fibers of the nerve. With supramaximal stimulation, the antidromic (travels in the opposite direction of normal conduction) motor pathway response invades motor neurons in the ventral spinal cord gray matter, which are activated producing an orthodromic (travels in the direction of normal conduction) second motor response (F wave). However, with less than supramaximal stimulation intensities, the activity traveling centrally along the sensory pathway activates reflex pathways in the spinal cord, which results in activation of the anterior horn cell and an EMG motor response, the H reflex. It is only as the stimulation intensity is increased that the H-reflex responses increase in amplitude and then decrease and eventually disappear, only to be replaced by F responses. H-reflex responses can be recorded from several muscles in the adult; however, the reflex is most often acquired from the gastrocnemius muscle following stimulation of the tibial nerve at the popliteal fossa (primarily via S1). In addition to monitoring the sensory and motor nerves, the H reflex also monitors the spinal cord gray matter at the level of the reflex. Since more cephalad spinal injury affects pathways that contribute to the excitability of the anterior horn cell, a more proximal spinal cord injury produces a block of the reflex at lower levels ("spinal shock").

APPLICATION OF THESE TECHNIQUES AND FUTURE DIRECTIONS

Based on the anatomy and physiology at risk during various surgical procedures, one or more of the previously discussed monitoring modalities can be used during surgery depending on the portions of the nervous system at risk. Application of these monitoring modalities can improve decision making and reduce injury.

PROCEDURES AFFECTING THE CEREBRAL CORTEX

CEREBRAL ISCHEMIA

A variety of monitoring techniques have been used when the procedure involves the cerebral cortex. As mentioned above, the ability to assess ischemia provides the opportunity to make corrections in the procedure or improve the neural environment (e.g., raise the blood pressure) to reduce risk. This has made monitoring useful with intracranial and extracranial vascular procedures.

The use of EEG monitoring for carotid endarterectomies (CEAs) done under general anesthesia is the standard

at many centers.[20] When ischemic changes occur that do not rapidly respond to increases in blood pressure, shunt placement is considered. Since the use of a shunt increases the risk of embolic stroke, EEG can assist in determining when shunt placement is not indicated and thus avoids the risk of unnecessary use and the production of emboli. In addition, the time interval between cross-clamping and EEG changes has also been used to estimate the allowable time without a shunt.[21] In one study in which 658 patients were monitored with EEG during cross-clamping, EEG changes indicative of ischemia were associated with an increased risk of ischemic stroke.[22] It is important to note that two thirds of the strokes were focal in nature and resulted from embolic events that may not have been detected by EEG monitoring.

Since EEG only monitors the electrical activity from the surface of the brain, the use of other monitoring techniques such as SSEPs may be helpful adjuncts to identify subcortical ischemia. SSEP monitoring has also been used during CEA for making decisions regarding shunt placement, to guide blood pressure management, and to predict postoperative morbidity. In some respects, the use of EEG and SSEPs are complementary as SSEPs are able to detect ischemia in deep cortical structures while EEG assesses a wider area of the cortical surface.[23] Meta-analysis of the combined use of EEG and SSEP monitoring suggests that when these two monitoring modalities are used together, they are effective in identifying ischemia and improving neurologic outcomes.[7]

EEG, SSEPs, and, more recently, MEPs have also been used for the detection of cerebral ischemia during surgical procedures involving intracranial arteries, aneurysms, and arteriovenous malformations (AVMs). They have also been used with interventional procedures for carotid artery angioplasty and deliberate occlusion of various arterial vessels, including aneurysms and AVMs.[24] When the cortical tissue at risk is involved in mediating the SSEP responses, SSEPs appear more sensitive than EEG for detecting cerebral ischemia in the sensory cortex. This is particularly true when the ischemia includes subcortical areas not monitored by EEG.[25] One neurosurgeon has concluded that "in principle, [the use of] SSEP monitoring makes sense with virtually all supratentorial procedures with regard to possible systemic or remote events, even if the somatosensory system is not involved."[26]

The primary use of SSEP monitoring during supratentorial surgery is for aneurysms of the anterior circulation where an improved outcome with their use as opposed to without has been observed.[27] For anterior cerebral artery (ACA) aneurysms, lower extremity SSEPs are more useful than upper extremity SSEPs because these arteries provide the blood supply to the cortical sensory areas for the lower extremities. However, upper extremity SSEPs may be useful if perforating arteries are at risk. Surgery involving middle cerebral artery circulation is best monitored by the use of upper extremity SSEPs. The use of upper extremity SSEPs is also preferred for aneurysms of the internal carotid arteries unless the aneurysms are at the carotid bifurcation. Here the presence of perforators makes the additional use of lower extremity SSEPs important. The author of one study involving the use of SSEP monitoring for aneurysm surgery stated that their use resulted in changes in 11.3% of these surgeries; the author now finds their use indispensable.[27]

During aneurysm surgery, SSEPs have been used to detect ischemia resulting from inadvertent, partial, or complete vessel occlusion; vasospasm; retractor pressure; suboptimal vessel clip application; and relative hypotension. Their use has resulted in changes of surgical technique, including stopping coagulation or dissection, applying papaverine, and changing the area and style of dissection.[26] They have also been used to assess the tolerance of the brain to temporary clipping; a very prompt loss of cortical SSEP responses (less than one minute after clipping) is associated with the development of a neurologic deficit if the clip remains in place. However, a delayed loss with prompt recovery after release of the clip is associated with the presence of collateral circulation and a markedly reduced incidence of neural morbidity. Symon et al. have suggested that when the N_{20} of the median nerve SSEP disappears slowly (over 4 minutes), 10 additional minutes of occlusion can be safely tolerated.[28]

Since multiple vascular territories can be affected during aneurysm and AVM procedures, the use of MEP in addition to EEG and SSEP monitoring can aid in the detection of ischemia and should be considered. MEP monitoring is particularly important during intracranial aneurysm surgery where perforating arteries affect the functional status of deep structures, including the motor pathways in the corona radiata, internal capsule, cerebral peduncle, basis pontis, and pyramids.[8] MEP monitoring is also important during resection or embolization of AVMs located near the central region or close to the sensory-motor pathways. Here the results of test occlusion of AVM feeders can be assessed for the functional compromise of nearby normal tissue before permanent manipulation occurs.

The use of MEP monitoring has been reported to be a means for identifying vasospasm and incorrect or inadequate aneurysm clip placement.[29] Similar correlations of MEP monitoring with outcomes has been seen with aneurysm clipping in the basilar, carotid, and middle cerebral circulations. Monitoring with MEPs is also valuable

during vascular surgery involving deep brain and brainstem structures near the motor pathways. Studies have found that when MEPs are acquired as often as every minute, they are more effective than SSEPs and EEG at detecting inadequate perfusion.[30]

SSEP and MEP monitoring have also been used for other procedures involving cerebral arteries. For example, SSEP monitoring has been used during neuroradiologic procedures such as carotid artery angioplasty, deliberate occlusion of various arterial vessels including aneurysms and AVMs, and streptokinase dissolution of blood clots.[24] It has also been found to be useful during occlusion of vessels in surgical procedures for the treatment of AVMs and cavernous malformations in the pericentral region of the brain. With AVMs, the use of monitoring has allowed provocative testing of the vascular supply in order to determine the safety of vessel sacrifice. In this case, test clamping or the injection of sodium amytal, which blocks the gray matter neural activity of MEPs, and lidocaine, which blocks the white matter conduction of SSEPs or MEPs, helps identify when the vascular supply to lesions involves critical pathways.[31]

METABOLIC SUPPRESSION TO REDUCE ISCHEMIC INJURY AND IDENTIFICATION OF CORTICAL SEIZURES

Because of the relationship between EEG and metabolism, EEG has been used to titrate the administration of barbiturates or other medications when intentional metabolic suppression of synaptic function is desired in order to improve the tolerance of the brain to ischemia (e.g., "brain protection"). This has been used when the vascular supply is compromised and when other maneuvers are unable to provide adequate cerebral blood flow (e.g., with temporary aneurysm clipping, surgery on the proximal aorta). The ability of EEG to detect seizures has made it indispensable for localization of seizure foci before resection or for identification of seizures when brain stimulation is used to identify areas such as the motor cortex or is used to produce temporary interruption of function (such as the interruption of speech used in an awake craniotomy to identify the eloquent regions of speech).

MAPPING OF THE SENSORY AND MOTOR CORTEX

SSEPs have been termed "indispensable" for localization of the sulcus, which demarcates the border between the sensory and motor cortex in the anesthetized patient.[32] Localization is accomplished by recording the cortical component of the median nerve SSEP using multicontact recording strips placed on the cortical surface. The central sulcus, separating the motor and sensory areas, is identified by a phase reversal of the responses, probably due to the horizontal nature of the dipole generator located in the gyrus.[33] In most instances, this technique, called sensory mapping, provides a means of identifying the sensory and motor cortex of patients, and its use can help the surgeon minimize injury to the motor cortex and provide a safe approach for the removal of tumors located below the cortical surface.[26,33]

However, in some instances, the anatomy of the cortical surface may be distorted by the presence of a tumor. In these instances, direct cortical stimulation (called motor mapping) may be used to elicit motor responses that can be visualized, or EMG responses (evoked or triggered EMG) can be recorded from various muscle groups in the limbs, face, and trunk. Stimulation of the cortical surface near the lesion will provide a means to assess what muscle groups to focus on, then recording electrodes can be placed within the appropriate musculature. Monitoring with both triggered EMG responses and SSEPs has been used during tumor removal near the motor cortex, motor tracts (including in the brainstem), and insula and also for cavernous angiomas.[26,29,34] With surgery near the motor cortex, direct motor cortex stimulation[35] has been successfully used to define the "edge" of the motor cortex and to limit undue motor injury with tumor resection.[30,36] In these cases the monitoring strategy is to continue resection until EMG responses are elicited at low-stimulation intensities. Although not all motor deficits can be avoided, the combined use of motor and sensory mapping is advocated to limit morbidity. For brain tumors, reversible MEP changes are usually associated with transient postoperative motor weakness. In these cases, the degree of MEP change correlates with the degree of postoperative paresis.[36,37]

PROCEDURES AFFECTING THE BRAINSTEM

CRANIAL NERVE MONITORING

Perhaps one of the most commonly used modalities during surgery in the brainstem is the use of spontaneous and evoked electromyography of the cranial nerves. The most common cranial nerve monitored during surgery is the facial nerve because of the frequent risk of facial nerve injury and the devastating impact of a postoperative paralysis. The muscles used for monitoring are the orbicularis oculi and orbicularis oris, ipsilateral to the surgery. Since the nerve may be intertwined

within brainstem tumors (e.g., acoustic neuroma), stimulation of the facial nerve enables location of the nerve in the operative site and warning of the unrecognized proximity of the nerve to operating instruments. During surgery, nonstimulated activity may warn of impending injury and change the surgical technique.

This monitoring is particularly helpful during removal of vestibular schwannomas (acoustic neuromas) when monitoring increases the likelihood that the anatomic integrity of the nerve will be maintained during surgery. In these cases, over 60% of patients with intact nerves at the conclusion of surgery will regain at least partial function several months postoperatively.[38] Reduction in the size of stimulated CMAPs of the facial nerve (CN VII) during posterior fossa surgery correlates with the immediate and long-term outcome of neurologic function.[39] For example, facial nerve monitoring during acoustic neuroma resection unequivocally reduces long-term postoperative facial nerve injury, leading to an improved quality of life and reduction in subsequent medical costs.[40]

Because of the improvement in outcome, an NIH consensus panel concluded, "The benefits of routine intraoperative monitoring of the facial nerve have been clearly established [in vestibular schwannoma]. This technique should be included in surgical therapy."[41] Therefore, facial nerve monitoring has become a standard of care in surgery for vestibular schwannoma and is commonly monitored in other surgeries in the cerebellopontine angle.

As described in Table 12.1, EMG monitoring can be used for all the cranial nerves with motor components. The oculomotor cranial nerves (CNs III, IV, and VI) are not commonly monitored, given the technical difficulties in placing recording needles, but may be of value during tumor removal in the region of the cavernous sinus or intraventricular tumors. In microvascular decompression for hemifacial spasm and trigeminal neuralgia, intraoperative stimulation of CNs V and VII both before and after isolation of a possible offending vessel has led to more accurate identification of offending vessels with better postoperative results.[42] EMG monitoring is useful during surgery involving cranial nerve compression syndromes, including trigeminal neuralgia (CN V) and vagoglossal-pharyngeal neuralgia (CNs IX and X).[9] Damage to lower cranial nerve nuclei (CNs IX–XII) can lead to complications of dyspnea and severe dysphagia, and aspiration requiring tracheostomy. Monitoring has been useful in auditory implant procedures and skull base surgery.

During surgery involving tumors of the posterior fossa, EMG monitoring helps to predict and possibly improve postoperative neurologic outcome. In a study of pediatric patients undergoing surgery for removal of tumors located in the brainstem where the lower cranial nerves (CNs IX, X, XII) were monitored, persistent neurotonic activity in a muscle innervated by one nerve resulted in a postoperative deficit in 73% of patients, and temporary increases in EMG activity associated with all three nerves was always accompanied by a deficit.[43] Postoperative aspiration pneumonia or the need for a tracheotomy was always associated with intraoperative EMG activity that arose from at least one of these cranial nerves.

MONITORING THE AUDITORY PATHWAY

Auditory brainstem responses (ABRs) are useful for hearing preservation during posterior fossa surgery for the removal of tumors because of the frequent involvement of the cochlear nerve with tumors in this region.[9,38] In general, if waves I and V are preserved during surgery, hearing is usually preserved, but if they are both lost, there is little chance of preservation of hearing postoperatively. In particular, ABR monitoring during the surgical removal of acoustic neuromas reduces the risk of damage to the acoustic nerve and improves the probability of postoperative hearing.

GENERAL VIABILITY OF THE BRAINSTEM

Since both the SSEPs and MEPs traverse the brainstem, they have been used to monitor its viability. ABR monitoring has been used during decompression of space-occupying lesions in the cerebellum, removal of cerebellar vascular malformations, and microvascular decompression for relief of hemifacial spasm or trigeminal neuralgia. SSEPs have been used during brainstem surgery to identify circumstances in which mechanical or vascular compromise of the brainstem is occurring near the surgical site or as a result of retractor placement. When both SSEPs and ABRs are used in combination, these techniques can be used to monitor the functional integrity of about 20% of the brainstem.

MEP monitoring is also a valuable monitoring technique to use during vascular surgery involving deep brain and brainstem structures near the motor pathways. Studies have found that the use of MEPs produced by direct cortical stimulation can be more effective than that of SSEPs or EEG at detecting inadequate perfusion.[26] Likewise, MEPs can be used to assess the general integrity of brainstem structures. Monitoring MEPs of the face and hand musculature can aid in assessing the corticospinal and corticobulbar tracts, particularly for tumors in the posterior fossa.[44]

With surgery close to the cerebral peduncles or the ventral medulla, injury to the corticospinal tracts is a concern, and monitoring with MEPs is important.[45,46] Brainstem motor mapping of the corticospinal tract (CT) can be done by using a hand-held stimulator to stimulate various areas within the brainstem and by recording CMAPs from appropriate muscle groups.[44] This technique has been found helpful in surgery involving midbrain tumors or surgery near the cerebral peduncle and ventral medulla where the corticospinal tract is often distorted.[44]

MAPPING OF THE BRAINSTEM

Similar to supratentorial mapping, electrophysiological techniques have been used in the brainstem for localization of structures during surgery and to identify optimal surgical windows to deeper regions.[47] A variety of "safe" entry zones have been identified in relation to the location of selected cranial nerve nuclei. However, because the usual locations are based on anatomic landmarks that may become distorted by the growth of lesions, mapping techniques are critical. In these cases, electrical stimulation of the surface of the brainstem is used to locate the cranial nerve nuclei. These techniques are based on recording muscle activity following stimulation of cranial nerve motor nuclei—CNs VII, IX, X, and XII—located on the floor of the fourth ventricle.[44,48]

PROCEDURES AFFECTING THE SPINAL CORD

SPINAL COLUMN CORRECTIVE SURGERY

Perhaps the largest application of electrophysiological monitoring with respect to procedures affecting the spinal cord is to reduce the risk of loss of spinal cord function by identifying changes in function that result from either mechanical or ischemic insults. The current risks of neurologic complications in spinal surgery are not minimal (anterior cervical diskectomy 0.46%, scoliosis correction 0.25–3.2%, intramedullary spinal cord tumor surgery 23.8–65.4%), and an improvement in outcomes has been observed as the result of monitoring.[49]

SSEPs were first used for monitoring purposes in the 1970s and were found to be very effective during scoliosis surgery. Improved outcomes relating to motor pathway function were shown in animal studies[50] in which a simultaneous loss of cortical SSEP amplitude and clinical motor function was seen. The utility of SSEP monitoring for scoliosis spinal surgery was shown in an analysis conducted by the Scoliosis Research Society (SRS) and the European Spinal Deformities Society. They evaluated the results of SSEP monitoring during the correction of spinal deformity in 51,263 surgeries (scoliosis, kyphosis, fractures, and spondylolisthesis) performed by 173 surgeons.[51] The overall incidence of neurologic injury was 0.55% (1 in 182 cases), well below the 0.7–4% historical average incidence expected for such surgical procedures without SSEP monitoring. The incidence of a major neurologic injury without any significant SSEP change was 0.063% (about 1 case in 1500 procedures), indicating that the loss of motor function without significant SSEP changes was rare despite the fact that the SSEP is transmitted in the posterior columns; sensory pathways that mediate proprioception and vibration sense. The economic impact of monitoring was assessed by Nuwer and colleagues, who estimated that the cost of monitoring a sufficient number of cases to prevent one major, persistent neurologic deficit (200 cases) is small compared to the cost of lifelong medical care for the treatment of that deficit.[51,52] Other authors have conducted similar cost analyses and concluded that properly applied, monitoring is cost effective.[53]

Numerous other studies have demonstrated improvements in spinal surgery outcomes when monitoring is used. As a consequence, the SRS has published a position statement that virtually makes the utilization of monitoring a standard of care during axial skeletal and spinal cord procedures.[54] The statement concludes that "neurophysiological monitoring can assist in the early detection of complications and possibly prevent postoperative morbidity in patients undergoing operations on the spine." This was echoed in the British literature as well when it was stated, "Today, it is standard practice to conduct some form of monitoring when performing any spinal operation that is associated with a high risk of neurologic injury. Generally, operations are considered to carry such a risk when corrective forces are applied to the spine, the patient has pre-existing neurologic damage, the cord is being invaded, or an osteotomy or other procedure is being carried out in immediate juxtaposition to the cord."[55] Hence, SSEP monitoring has become commonplace during a wide variety of spinal surgical procedures.

Since the loss of posterior column SSEP responses correlates well with the loss of motor function mediated by more anteriorly located white matter and gray matter, it is likely that the Harrington rod distraction and derotation that was then used during scoliosis correction was producing an effect across the entire spinal cord (e.g., spinal ischemia). In order to detect the rare case when motor injury occurred in the absence of SSEP change, a better assessment of motor function was needed. As such, with the development of MEP monitoring, it became commonplace for MEPs to be acquired during spinal column surgery.

The potential dissociation of the neural function mediated by the motor and posterior column pathways was enhanced by the evolution of surgical procedures with sublaminar wires, hooks, screws, and a variety of other hardware devices that could produce focal injuries in the anterior spinal cord. This was particularly true when the operative procedure involved portions of the spinal cord, which included gray matter that can be monitored by the use of MEPs (e.g., levels above the cauda equina). Two recent studies examined outcomes and reported a high correlation of the results of MEP monitoring and outcomes. In the largest study, 11.3% of the patients had MEP changes; of the five patients with persistent MEP changes, all had permanent neurologic injury.[56] During cervical spine surgery, MEP monitoring is commonly used, as it is believed to decrease morbidity in part because it may allow differentiation between cervical cord myelopathy and peripheral neuropathy.[57]

It is important to note that monitoring has also been shown to detect unfavorable physiological circumstances. In particular, SSEPs have been shown to reflect the viability of the spinal cord during deliberate hypotension or deliberate hemodilution.[58] Levels of hypotension or anemia not usually associated with injury may, in a specific individual, cause neuronal damage and permanent injury if not corrected. Not surprisingly, one of the common maneuvers used during spinal surgery and deterioration of SSEP or MEP monitoring is an incremental increase in the patient's blood pressure.

The effectiveness of MEP monitoring is such that the Stagnara wake-up test is less commonly used. However, some surgeons, anesthesiologists, and intraoperative monitoring physicians (such as neurologists) believe that it remains the gold standard, and its use is still recommended by some for confirming possible injury when the monitoring techniques become persistently abnormal during a surgical procedure.[59] Some individuals monitor by using the H reflex as a supplement to the MEP or when they are unable to acquire MEPs. The degree of H-reflex suppression has been found to correlate with the degree of spinal injury. A sustained loss of the reflex or even a 90% amplitude decrease has been found to strongly correlate with the onset of a new motor deficit.[6]

INTRAMEDULLARY SPINAL CORD SURGERY

The potential for focal injury to the motor tracts is enhanced when the surgical procedure may compromise the anterior spinal artery or when the surgery is conducted within the spinal cord, such as operations for intramedullary abnormalities. Studies strongly suggest that the use of MEPs during intramedullary spinal cord tumor resection improves the likelihood of the preservation of long-term motor function.[44,48,60] Here, the MEP is the only reliable monitor of motor pathway function and is an earlier predictor of impending damage to the cord than the SSEP because of the more precarious nature of the blood supply to the motor tracts in the anterior spinal cord. Using an anterior approach for an intramedullary spinal cord tumor resection, focal injury to the anterior spinal vasculature or motor tracts is often not detected or is detected many minutes after injury when using SSEP monitoring alone.[8,61] MEP monitoring has been successfully used to define the "edge" of intramedullary spinal tumors and to maximize resection while minimizing motor impairment. When using MEPs for monitoring purposes, the descending volley of neural activity that is mediated by the motor pathways and which can be recorded directly from the surface of the spinal cord is known as a D wave. This volley eventually produces a muscle response as well. For specific identification of the motor tracts, stimulation within the spinal cord shortly after transcranial stimulation produces a "collision," which blocks the D wave or the muscle response, identifying the location of the tract.[62–64]

In these cases, monitoring of the D wave using an epidural electrode as well as recording of the CMAP can allow better correlation with motor outcome.[1] This is because the amplitude of the D wave is considered a semiquantitative assessment of the number of fast conducting fibers of the corticospinal tract and correlates better with long-term functional motor outcome than the muscle response (CMAP).[10,44] When the D-wave amplitude is unchanged or reduced less than 50%, the patient will have postoperative motor function, even if a temporary loss of a muscle response is seen. Transient postoperative paralysis, lasting several hours to days, is thought to be due to a loss of accessory motor pathways (e.g., propriospinal systems that facilitate the corticospinal pathway).[1] Since as little as 10% of the corticospinal tract fibers may be necessary for motor function, the warning criteria for D-wave changes is often 30–50% loss before surgery is halted or abandoned.[44]

Studies report an excellent correlation with monitoring and clinical outcome.[65] Using combined SSEP and MEP monitoring yields 100% sensitivity and 91% specificity for the detection of adverse outcomes from intramedullary spinal cord surgery.[44] With spinal AVMs, monitoring has allowed provocative testing of the vascular supply to determine the safety of vessel sacrifice. In this case, test clamping or the injection of sodium amytal, which blocks gray matter neural activity of MEP, and lidocaine, which blocks white matter conduction of the SSEP or MEP, helps to identify when the vascular supply to lesions involves critical pathways.[31] This is essentially a "Wada" test of the spinal cord and can be used to detect spinal cord ischemia as may occur from blockage of catheters used for injection (such as for selective cannulation during interventional radiology), vasospasm, and dissection or occlusion of a critical feeding vessel.

MAPPING THE SPINAL CORD MIDLINE

Electrophysiological monitoring can also be useful to assist the surgeon in finding a safe entry zone to enter the spinal cord for intramedullary surgery. In this case, the desired posterior approach is along the midline, between the dorsal column pathways. Unfortunately, the intramedullary abnormality may distort the midline, making this entry route unclear visually. Since SSEPs are mediated by the dorsal columns, which lie adjacent to the midline, stimulation of nerves in the lower extremities with recording of the resulting responses by means of a series of contacts across the posterior aspect of the cord provides a means for identifying the dorsal median sulcus.[64] This reduces the risk of iatrogenic injury to other regions of the spinal cord but may produce injury to the dorsal columns, rendering the SSEP less effective for monitoring.

MONITORING TO REDUCE SPINAL NERVE ROOT INJURY

During spine surgery, a radiculopathy may be caused by the unfavorable placement of instrumentation or when surgery involves a percutaneous approach to the spine traversing nerves or nerve plexi (e.g., transverse lumbar interbody fusion). A variety of muscles can be used for monitoring purposes depending on the specific nerve root(s) to be monitored (Table 12.2). Unfortunately, the SSEP is less effective for this monitoring as the nerves used by the SSEP are only a portion of the nerves potentially at risk, and when they do include the desired nerves, the transmission through an abnormal nerve root response can be masked by other normal nerve root responses, resulting in normal-appearing SSEP responses.[4] The MEP may also be less specific than EMG for individual nerve roots, as multiple nerve roots will be simultaneously activated by MEP monitoring, and muscles may be innervated through more than one nerve root such that problems in an individual nerve root may be masked.

EMG monitoring has achieved widespread usage as a means of reducing the risk of injury to nerve roots during placement of pedicle screws, where the risk of complications is as frequent as 15–25%.[66] EMG testing can be used to identify improper screw placement by stimulation of the pedicle screw or screw hole with a monopolar probe.

The current intensity that is needed to activate a nerve root (as seen by triggered EMG from a muscle innervated by that nerve root) correlates with the screw being contained within the pedicle (high current necessary to activate the EMG), having breached the pedicle wall (lower current), or having the screw threads near the spinal cord or nerve roots (very low current similar to the current needed for direct stimulation of the root).[67] Several case series and studies support the usefulness of this pedicle screw testing in reducing nerve root injury.[68–70]

SURGERY ON THE CAUDA EQUINA

The potential for nerve root injuries is also significant during surgery on the cauda equina. Procedures such as release of a tethered cord or tumor excision carry the risk of damage to nerve roots that innervate the muscles of the leg, anal muscle, and urethral sphincter. Damage to these nerve roots is extremely debilitating (especially loss of bowel and bladder control), and every effort is sought to avoid this complication. EMG monitoring is essential for differentiating neural from non-neural tissue by using stimulation methods of structures to determine if they can be resected.[71] As with many types of surgery, when monitoring tethered cord surgery, other monitoring techniques such as SSEPs and MEPs may also be used, but EMG techniques provide the best guide to the surgeon for tissue resection and untethering purposes.

DORSAL RHIZOTOMY

EMG techniques are also essential during dorsal rhizotomy surgery for the reduction of severe incapacitating spasticity (often the result of cerebral palsy). The spasticity is thought to be due to an imbalance of muscular innervation from hyperactivity of sensory nerve rootlets devoid of adequate supraspinal control. As such, the surgical approach is to remove some rootlets to restore the balance. EMG recording is used to identify the most hyperactive rootlets by observing the spread of activity to adjacent myotomes when the rootlets are stimulated (usually between L2 and S2).[44,72] The recording of EMG activity is also key to avoiding an injury to rootlets that innervate the anal sphincter and urogential system, so as to minimize bowel and bladder complications.

MAJOR VASCULAR PROCEDURES

The SSEP and MEP have been used during surgery when the vascular supply to the spinal cord may be compromised, resulting in ischemia of the spinal cord neural tracts. This can occur during corrective anterior thoracic spine surgery and during repair of thoracoabdominal aneurysms when interruption of the radicular perforators from the aorta (especially the Artery of Adamkiewicz) and the pelvic supply to the caudal spinal cord may place the spinal cord at risk for ischemia. Of particular interest are procedures involving the thoracoabdominal aorta, where the reported incidence of paraplegia varies from 0.5% with aortic coarctation repairs when the procedure is short and the patient usually has well-developed collateral circulation to nearly 48% with emergency repairs of extensive thoracoabdominal degenerative lesions.[73,74]

Early studies using SSEPs indicated that when a slow onset of cortical and subcortical SSEP changes occurred over a period of greater than 15 minutes, this was usually an indication of peripheral nerve ischemia. Isolated events, such as the femoral artery bypass cannula occluding flow to the leg, are some of the more frequent causes of peripheral nerve ischemia and unilateral loss of SSEPs. On the other hand, if bilateral SSEP changes occurred within a period of less than 15 minutes, it was assumed to be of spinal cord origin—either from inadequate distal aorta perfusion or loss of critical intercostals.[75] Thus, clinicians have used SSEP monitoring to determine if a bypass (e.g. atrial-femoral bypass) was necessary, if the blood pressure within the bypass was adequate, and if it was safe to exclude or remove a specific radicular artery. SSEPs have been shown to be restored when critical intercostals vessels are reimplanted or unclamped. Rapid reperfusion of critical intercostal vessels restores the monitored SSEPs and appears to reduce the risk of paraplegia.[76]

However, like spinal column surgery, the results of SSEP monitoring often correlate with motor injury but can miss some motor tract injuries.[77] The correlation was best when the SSEP loss occurred rapidly after cross-clamping (within 3–5 minutes) or when the duration of SSEP loss was prolonged (40–60 minutes).[75,76] The MEP has been used to more specifically monitor motor tract function during surgical or interventional treatment for thoracoabdominal aneurysms.[78] Use of MEP monitoring allows for rapid detection of ischemia because the gray matter, with its high metabolic rate, is more sensitive to ischemia than the white matter tracts, which mediate the SSEP or MEP.[78] All studies, both clinical and experimental, have reported a rapid change in MEP, within 2–4 minutes, attributable to ischemic conditions. This rapid response provides more useful feedback in the intraoperative environment where time is critical in determining outcome. Although false-negative results with MEP monitoring have occurred (i.e., immediate postoperative paralysis with preserved intraoperative MEPs), most studies have shown an excellent correlation of outcome with MEP findings.[77,79] In these procedures, monitoring has been used to guide management of blood flow to the brain or metabolic suppression when the aortic arch is involved (EEG, cortical SSEP) and to guide maneuvers such as the drainage of cerebrospinal fluid that are used to improve spinal cord perfusion pressure.

PROCEDURES AFFECTING THE PERIPHERAL NERVES OR PLEXI

Since the SSEP and MEP traverse peripheral nerves and plexi, these techniques have the potential to monitor during several types of procedures where the peripheral nerve is at risk. For example, monitoring cranial nerve function for surgery outside the brainstem is also useful. Monitoring recurrent laryngeal and superior laryngeal branches of the vagus nerve (CN X) is often used in neck dissections and thyroid removal, for which the reported incidence of recurrent laryngeal nerve injury is 2.3–5.2%.[80] In these cases EMG monitoring is performed by placing needle electrodes in the cricothyroid or vocalis muscles or by the use of contact electrodes on an endotracheal tube. It has been particularly useful with malignancy, neck re-exploration for hemorrhage, second operations, and anatomic distortion from radiation. Similar techniques are used during anterior cervical spine fusions, radical neck dissection, and parotid and facial surgery using several cranial nerves (CNs VII, X, XI).

Monitoring has also been useful to assess the integrity of peripheral nerves. For example, SSEP monitoring can aid in detecting potential nerve injury related to arm positioning, which is usually a stretch or pressure injury. Ulnar nerve injury, thought to be as high as 4.8% in the prone position, can be detected by recording the response to ulnar nerve stimulation in the wrist or forearm.[65] Similarly, EMG monitoring has been used to guide lower extremity limb lengthening and to avoid sciatic nerve injury during hip arthroplasty or arthroscopy.[81]

Finally, when approaching a neuroma in continuity, the outcome is improved when removal of the neuroma and reapproximation of the nerve is done only when there is no neural continuity in the neuroma. The assessment of this continuity is done by stimulating the nerve on one side of the injury and observing whether a response is present on the other side. The presence of an evoked action potential indicates that some continuity is present and regeneration is occurring such that the best outcome will occur without

surgical repair. If the injury is proximal, such as a nerve root avulsion, the evoked response must be recorded centrally as with the SSEP or DEP.[4] If the injury is very distal, continuity may be assessed by recording the muscle EMG from stimulation similar to stimulated EMG or MEP. Finally, if an injury has occurred within a plexus (such as a brachial plexus trauma), these techniques can be used to locate the abnormality within the plexus by identifying the anatomic location of disrupted electrical continuity.[82]

CONCLUSION

The use of electrophysiological mapping and monitoring techniques has become commonplace during various neurosurgical procedures, and they are used in order to improve surgical decision making. Longitudinal studies comparing outcomes of patients having intraoperative monitoring with retrospective nonmonitored controls has been used to meet "evidence-based" principles.[83] As such, in many institutions neurophysiological monitoring has become a standard of care during axial skeletal,[83–85] head and neck,[86] base of skull, or posterior fossa surgery[42,87] and is increasingly being explored for use during intracranial aneurysm clipping, tumor resection,[30,34,88] and hip arthroplasty.[81]

Typically, multiple techniques are used together to increase the utility of the monitoring. For example, SSEPs, EMG activity, and MEPs are frequently combined for spinal surgery monitoring purposes. In addition to helping guide the surgical procedure, these techniques may assist in reducing neural morbidity by guiding the physiological management (notably blood pressure management) to a better outcome when complete or timely reversal of the procedural insult, such as aneurysm clip reconstruction, is not possible. Expanded use of intraoperative monitoring modalities may be an important step toward reducing the incidence of the neurologic complications of surgery and anesthesia.

CONFLICT OF INTEREST STATEMENT

A.K., T.S., and R.T. have no financial conflicts of interest to disclose.

REFERENCES

1. Deletis V. Intraoperative neurophysiology and methodologies used to monitor the functional integrity of the motor system. In: Deletis V, Shils JL, eds. *Neurophysiology in Neurosurgery*. New York: Academic Press, 2002:25.

2. Harper CM, Daube JR. Facial nerve electromyography and other cranial nerve monitoring [see comment]. *J Clin Neurophysiol.* 1998;15:206.

3. Harper CM. Intraoperative cranial nerve monitoring: *Muscle Nerve.* 2004;29:339.

4. Holland NR. Intraoperative electromyography. *J Clin Neurophysiol.* 2002;19:444.

5. Kothbauer KF, Novak K. Intraoperative monitoring for tethered cord surgery: an update: *Neurosurgery.* 2004;16:E8.

6. Leppanen RE. Intraoperative applications of the H-reflex and F-response: a tutorial. *J Clin. Monit Comput.* 2006;20:267.

7. Lopez JR. The use of evoked potentials in intraoperative neurophysiologic monitoring. *Phys Med Rehabil Clin N Am.* 2004;15:63.

8. Macdonald DB. Intraoperative motor evoked potential monitoring: overview and update: *J Clin Monit Comput.* 2006;20:347.

9. Moller A. *Intraoperative Neurophysiological Monitoring.* New York: Springer, 2011.

10. Sala F, Krzan MJ, Deletis V, et al. Intraoperative neurophysiological monitoring in pediatric neurosurgery: why, when, how? *Childs Nerv Syst.* 2002;18:264.

11. Shils JL, Tagliati M, Alterman RL. Neurophysiological monitoring during neurosurgery for movement disorders. In: Deletis V, Shils JL, eds. *Neurophysiology in Neurosurgery.* Boston: Academic Press; 2002:405.

12. Jameson LC, Sloan TB. Monitoring of the brain and spinal cord. *Anesthesiol Clin.* 2006;24:777.

13. Jameson LC, Sloan TB. Using EEG to monitor anesthesia drug effects during surgery: *J Clin Monit Comput.* 2006;20:445.

14. Sloan T, Jameson LC. Monitoring anesthetic effect. In: Koht A, Sloan T, Toleikis JR, eds. *Monitoring the Nervous System for Anesthesiologists and other Health Care Professionals.* New York: Springer; 2012:337.

15. MacDonald DB, Pillay N. Intraoperative electrocorticography in temporal lobe epilepsy surgery: *Canadian Journal of Neurological Sciences.* 2000;27 Suppl 1:S85,

16. Prass RL, Kinney SE, Hardy Jr RW, et al. Acoustic (loudspeaker) facial EMG monitoring: II. Use of evoked EMG activity during acoustic neuroma resection. *Otolaryngol Head Neck Surg.* 1987;97:541.

17. Jameson LC, Janik DJ, Sloan TB. Electrophysiologic monitoring in neurosurgery. *Anesthesiol Clin.* 2007;25:605.

18. Aravabhumi S, Izzo KL, Bakst BL. Brainstem auditory evoked potentials: intraoperative monitoring technique in surgery of posterior fossa tumors: *Arch Phys Med Rehab.* 1987;68:142.

19. Angelo R, Moller AR. Contralateral evoked brainstem auditory potentials as an indicator of intraoperative brainstem manipulation in cerebellopontine angle tumors. *Neurol Res.* 1996;18:528.

20. Findlay JM, Marchak BE, Pelz DM, et al. Carotid endarterectomy: a review. *Can J Neurol Sci.* 2004;31:22.

21. Deriu GP, Milite D, Mellone G, et al. Clamping ischemia, threshold ischemia and delayed insertion of the shunt during carotid endarterectomy with patch. *J Cardiovasc Surg.* 1999;40:249.

22. Krul JM, van Gijn J, Ackerstaff RG, et al. Site and pathogenesis of infarcts associated with carotid endarterectomy. *Stroke.* 1989;20:324.

23. Lam AM, Manninen PH, Ferguson GG, et al. Monitoring electrophysiologic function during carotid endarterectomy: a comparison of somatosensory evoked potentials and conventional electroencephalogram. *Anesthesiology.* 1991;75:15.

24. Dietz A, von Kummer R, Adams HP. Balloon occlusion test of the internal carotid artery for evaluating resectability of blood vessel infiltrating cervical metastasis of advanced head and neck cancers: Heidelberg experience. *Laryngorhinootologie.* 1993;72:558.

25. Ragazzoni A, Chiaramonit R, Zaccara G, et al. Simultaneous monitoring of multichannel somatosensory evoked potentials and electroencephalogrm during carotid endarterectomy: a comparison of the two methods to detect cerbral ischemia. *Clin Neurophysiol.* 2000;111:S138.

26. Neuloh G, Schramm J. Intraoperative neurophysiological mapping and monitoring for supratentorial procedures. In: Deletis V, Shils JL, eds. *Neurophysiology and Neurosurgery.* New York: Academic Press; 2002:339.

27. Schramm J, Zentner J, Pechstein U. Intraoperative SEP monitoring in aneurysm surgery. *Neurol Res.* 1994;16:20.

28. Symon L, Momma F, Murota T. Assessment of reversible cerebral ischaemia in man: intraoperative monitoring of the somatosensory evoked response. *Acta Neurochir Suppl* (Wien). 1988;42:3.

29. Szelenyi A, Langer D, Kothbauer K, et al. Monitoring of muscle motor evoked potentials during cerebral aneurysm surgery: intraoperative changes and postoperative outcome. *J Neurosurg.* 2006;105:675.

30. Neuloh G, Pechstein U, Cedzich C, et al. Motor evoked potential monitoring with supratentorial surgery. *Neurosurgery.* 2004;54:1061.

31. Guerit JM. Neuromonitoring in the operating room: why, when, and how to monitor? *Electroencephalogr Clin Neurophysiol.* 1998;106:1.

32. Firsching R, Klug N, Borner U, et al. Lesions of the sensorimotor region: somatosensory evoked potentials and ultrasound guided surgery. *Acta Neurochir* (Wien). 1992;118:87.

33. Cedzich C, Taniguchi M, Schafer S, et al. Somatosensory evoked potential phase reversal and direct motor cortex stimulation during surgery in and around the central region. *Neurosurgery.* 1996;38:962.

34. Neuloh G, Schramm J. Monitoring of motor evoked potentials compared with somatosensory evoked potentials and microvascular Doppler ultrasonography in cerebral aneurysm surgery. *J Neurosurg.* 2004;100:389.

35. Neuloh G, Schramm J. Motor evoked potential monitoring for the surgery of brain tumours and vascular malformations. *Adv Tech Stand Neurosurg.* 2004;29:171.

36. Mikuni N, Okada T, Enatsu R, et al. Clinical impact of integrated functional neuronavigation and subcortical electrical stimulation to preserve motor function during resection of brain tumors. *J Neurosurg.* 2007;106:593,

37. Zhou H, Kelly P. Transcranial electrical motor evoked potential monitoring for brain tumor resection. *Neurosurgery.* 2001;48:1075.

38. Yingling C, Ashram YA. Intraoperative monitoring of cranial nerves in skull base surgery. In: Jackler RK, Brackmann D, eds. *Neurotology.* 2nd ed. Philadelphia: Elsevier-Mosby; 2005:258.

39. Harner SG, Daube JR, Ebersold MJ, et al. Improved preservation of facial nerve function with use of electrical monitoring during removal of acoustic neuromas. *Mayo Clin Proc.* 1987;62:92.

40. Wilson L, Lin E, Lalwani A. Cost-effectiveness of intraoperative facial nerve monitoring in middle ear or mastoid surgery. *Laryngoscope.* 2003;113:412.

41. National Institutes of Health (NIH). Consensus statement. 9. Consensus Development Conference, December 11–13, 1991.

42. Mooij JJA, Mustafa MK, van Weerden TW. Hemifacial spasm: intraoperative electromyographic monitoring as a guide for microvascular decompression. *Neurosurgery.* 2001;49:1365.

43. Glasker S, Pechstein U, Vougioukas VI, et al. Monitoring motor function during resection of tumours in the lower brain stem and fourth ventricle. *Childs Nerv Syst.* 2006;22:1288.

44. Sala F, Lanteri P, Bricolo A. Motor evoked potential monitoring for spinal cord and brain stem surgery. *Adv Tech Stand Neurosurg.* 2004;29:133.

45. Deletis V, Sala F, Morota N. Intraoperative neurophysiological monitoring and mapping during brainstem surgery: a modern approach. *Operat Tech Neurosurg.* 2000;3:109.

46. Deletis V, Kothbauer KF. Intraoperative neurophysiology of the corticospinal tract. In: Stalberg E, Sharma HS, Olsson Y, eds. *Spinal Cord Monitoring.* New York: Springer; 1998:421.

47. Bricolo A, Sala F. Surgery of brainstem lesions. In: Deletis V, Shils JL, eds. *Neurophysiology in Neurosurgery.* Boston: Academic Press; 2002:267.

48. Morota N, Deletis V, Epstein FJ. Brainstem mapping. In: Deletis V, Shils JL, eds. *Neurophysiology in Neurosurgery.* Boston: Academic Press; 2002:319.

49. Costa P, Bruno A, Bonzanino M, et al. Somatosensory- and motor-evoked potential monitoring during spine and spinal cord surgery. *Spinal Cord*. 2007;45:86.

50. Croft TJ, Brodkey JS, Nulsen FE, et al. Reversible spinal cord trauma: a model for electrical monitoring of spinal cord function. *J Neurosurg*. 1972;36:402.

51. Nuwer MR, Dawson EG, Carlson LG, et al. Somatosensory evoked potential spinal cord monitoring reduces neurologic deficits after scoliosis surgery: results of a large multicenter survey. *Electroencephalogr Clin Neurophysiol*. 1995;96:6.

52. Nuwer MR. Spinal cord monitoring with somatosensory techniques. *J Clin Neurophysiol*. 1998;15:183.

53. Owen J. Cost efficacy of intraoperative monitoring. *Semin Spine Surg*. 1997;9:348.

54. Scoliosis Research Society. Position statement on somatosensory evoked potential monitoring of neurologic spinal cord function during surgery. Park Ridge, Illinois; 1992.

55. Loughman BA, Fennelly ME, Henley M, et al. The effects of differing concentrations of bupivacaine on the epidural somatosensory evoked potential after posterior tibial nerve stimulation. *Anesth Analg*. 1995;81:147.

56. Langeloo DD, Lelivelt A, Louis Journee H, et al. Transcranial electrical motor-evoked potential monitoring during surgery for spinal deformity: a study of 145 patients. *Spine*. 2003;28:1043.

57. Christakos A. The value of motor and somatosensory evoked potentials in evaluation of cervical myelopathy in the presence of peripheral neuropathy. *Spine* 2004;29:e239–247.

58. Grundy BL. Intraoperative monitoring of sensory-evoked potentials. *Anesthesiology*. 1983;58:72.

59. Papastefanou SL, Henderson LM, Smith NJ, et al. Surface electrode somatosensory-evoked potentials in spinal surgery: implications for indications and practice. *Spine*. 2000;25:2467.

60. Sala F, Palandri G, Basso E, et al. Motor evoked potential monitoring improves outcome after surgery for intramedullary spinal cord tumors: a historical control study. *Neurosurgery*. 2006;58:1129.

61. Pelosi L, Lamb J, Grevitt M, et al. Combined monitoring of motor and somatosensory evoked potentials in orthopaedic spinal surgery. *Clin. Neurophysiol*. 2002;113:1082.

62. Quinones-Hinojosa A, Gulati M, Lyon R, et al. Spinal cord mapping as an adjunct for resection of intramedullary tumors: surgical technique with case illustrations. *Neurosurgery*. 2002;51:1199.

63. Deletis V. Intraoperative neurophysiology of the corticospinal tract of the spinal cord. *Suppl Clin Neurophysiol*. 2006;59:107.

64. Deletis V, Bueno De Camargo A. Interventional neurophysiological mapping during spinal cord procedures. *Stereotact Funct Neurosurg*. 2001;77:25,

65. Lorenzini NA, Schneider JH. Temporary loss of intraoperative motor-evoked potential and permanent loss of somatosensory-evoked potentials associated with a postoperative sensory deficit. *J Neurosurg Anesthesiol*. 1996;8:142.

66. Calancie B, Madsen P, Lebwohl N. Stimulus-evoked EMG monitoring during transpedicular lumbosacral spine instrumentation. Initial clinical results. *Spine*. 1994;19:2780.

67. Toleikis JR. Neurophysiological monitoring during pedicle screw placement. In: Deletis V, Shils JL, eds. *Neurophysiology in Neurosurgery*. New York: Academic Press; 2002:231.

68. Reidy DP, Houlden D, Nolan PC, et al. Evaluation of electromyographic monitoring during insertion of thoracic pedicle screws. *J Bone Joint Surg Br*. 2001;83:1009.

69. Bose B, Wierzbowski LR, Sestokas AK, et al. Neurophysiologic monitoring of spinal nerve root function during instrumented posterior lumbar spine surgery. *Spine*. 2002;27:1444.

70. Krassioukov AV, Sarjeant R, Arkia H, et al. Multimodality intraoperative monitoring during complex lumbosacral procedures: indications, techniques, and long-term follow-up review of 61 consecutive cases [see comment]. *J Neurosurg Spine*. 2004;1:243.

71. Quinones-Hinojosa A, Gadkary CA, Gulati M, et al. Neurophysiological monitoring for safe surgical tethered cord syndrome release in adults. *Surg Neurol*. 2004;62:127.

72. Abbott R. Sensory rhizotomy for the treatment of childhood spasticity. In: Deletis V, Shils JL, eds. *Neurophysiology in Neurosurgery*. Boston: Academic Press; 2002:219.

73. Connolly JE. Hume memorial lecture. Prevention of spinal cord complications in aortic surgery. *Am J Surg*. 1998;176:92.

74. Crawford ES, Crawford JL, Safi HJ, et al. Thoracoabdominal aortic aneurysms: preoperative and intraoperative factors determining immediate and long-term results of operations in 605 patients: *Journal of Vascular Surgery*. 1986;3:389,

75. Robertazzi RR, Cunningham JN, Jr. Monitoring of somatosensory evoked potentials: a primer on the intraoperative detection of spinal cord ischemia during aortic reconstructive surgery. *Semin Thorac Cardiovasc Surg*. 1998;10:11.

76. Laschinger JC, Izumoto H, Kouchoukos NT. Evolving concepts in prevention of spinal cord injury during operations on the descending thoracic and thoracoabdominal aorta. *Ann Thorac Surg*. 1987;44:667.

77. de Haan P, Kalkman CJ. Spinal cord monitoring: somatosensory- and motor-evoked potentials. *Anesthesiol Clin North Am*. 2001;19:923.

78. Sloan TB, Jameson LC. Electrophysiologic monitoring during surgery to repair the thoraco-abdominal aorta. *J Clin Neurophysiol*. 2007;24:316.

79. Dong CCJ, MacDonald DB, Janusz MT. Intraoperative spinal cord monitoring during descending thoracic and thoracoabdominal aneurysm surgery. *Ann Thorac Surg*. 2002;74:S1873.

80. Pearlman RC, Isley MR, Ruben GD, et al. Intraoperative monitoring of the recurrent laryngeal nerve using acoustic, free-run, and evoked electromyography. *J Clin Neurophysiol*. 2005;22:148.

81. Brown DM, McGinnis WC, Mesghali H. Neurophysiologic intraoperative monitoring during revision total hip arthroplasty. *J Bone Joint Surg Am*. 2002;84-A(Suppl 2):56,

82. Crum BA, Strommen JA. Peripheral nerve stimulation and monitoring during operative procedures. *Muscle Nerve*. 2007;35:159.

83. Forbes HJ, Allen PW, Waller CS, et al. Spinal cord monitoring in scoliosis surgery. Experience with 1168 cases. *J Bone Joint Surg Br*. 1991;73:487.

84. Toleikis JR. Intraoperative monitoring using somatosensory evoked potentials. A position statement by the American Society of Neurophysiological Monitoring. *J Clin Monit Comput*. 2005;19:241.

85. Padberg A, Wilson-Holden T, Lenke LG, Bridwell KH. Somatosenory and motor-evoked potential monitoring without a wake-up test during idiopathic scoliosis surgery: an accepted standard of care. *Spine*. 1998;23:1392.

86. Edwards BM, Kileny PR. Intraoperative neurophysiologic monitoring: indications and techniques for common procedures in otolaryngology–head and neck surgery. *Otolaryngol Clin North Am*. 2005;38:631.

87. Freye E, Levy JV. Cerebral monitoring in the operating room and the intensive care unit: an introductory for the clinician and a guide for the novice wanting to open a window to the brain. Part I: The electroencephalogram. *J Clin Monit Comput*. 2005;19:1.

88. Quinones-Hinojosa A, Lyon R, Zada G, et al. Changes in transcranial motor evoked potentials during intramedullary spinal cord tumor resection correlate with postoperative motor function. *Neurosurgery*. 2005;56:982.

89. Jameson LC, Sloan TB. Monitoring of the brain and spinal cord. *Anesthesiology Clin*. 2006;24:777.

13.

NEUROLOGIC BIOMARKERS

Juan P. Cata

INTRODUCTION

Biomarkers are molecules released by a variety of cells in the human body in response to damage or significant change in function. Perhaps the most understood and used biomarkers in the perioperative setting are the cardiac troponins. Troponins have two essential characteristics: prognostic and predictive value. Similarly, neurologic biomarkers with prognostic capabilities can be used to identify patients at risk of suffering neurologic damage and show response after a specific therapy is given to ameliorate a neurologic insult.[1]

Biomarkers can be classified according to the aspect of injury they reflect: susceptibility, effect, and exposure. Susceptibility biomarkers are used to identify patients with a genetically mediated predisposition to a specific condition (e.g., ApoE). Effect biomarkers measure early biological effects, such as structural or functional changes in affected cells or tissues, or actual clinical diseases (e.g., S100B, Tau protein, neuron-specific enolase). Exposure biomarkers are employed to measure the actual chemicals, or chemical metabolites, and can be measured to determine different characteristics of a patient's exposure (carboxyhemoglobin).[2] Other characteristics of central nervous system (CNS) markers should include 1) easy detection in the blood, urine, or cerebrospinal fluid (CSF); 2) resistance to cytoplasmatic and extracellular proteolytic activity; 3) nonrenal excretion; and 4) affordability.

Delirium, stroke, postoperative cognitive dysfunction (POCD), spinal cord ischemia, and sepsis-associated encephalopathy are among the most devastating perioperative neurologic complications. There is increasing interest in identifying neurologic biomarkers that are sensitive and specific enough to make an early and precise diagnosis of any of these perioperative complications before they progress or become irreversible. Unfortunately, however, no consensus exists on which biomarker is the brain "troponin" to detect CNS insult. Perhaps more disturbing is the fact that there are no simple and cost-efficient modalities available to measure CNS reserve. It is also important to note that the currently studied neurobiomarkers cannot differentiate between focal CNS insult (stroke or spinal cord injury) and global neurologic insult (sepsis and post–cardiopulmonary bypass) (Figure 13.1).

In this chapter, we will present the evidence concerning neurologic biomarkers in the perioperative period: S100B protein, neuron-specific enolase (NSE), Tau protein, the metalloproteinases, and ubiquitin C-terminal hydroxylase-L1.

S100B PROTEIN

GENERAL CONCEPTS

The S100B protein is a homodimeric protein that belongs to the family of Ca^{2+}-Zn^{2+}-mediated proteins (S100 proteins).[3] The S100B dimer was thought to be specific to the

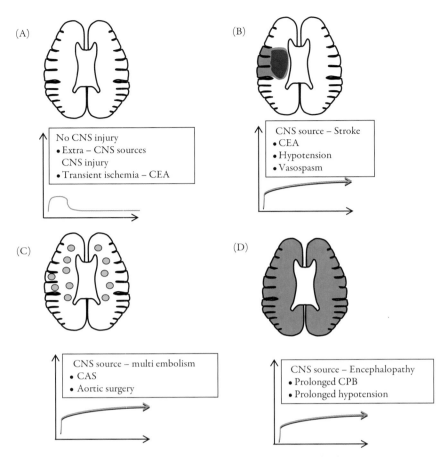

Figure 13.1 This figure shows the different type of CNS injury: (**A**) minimal or transient injury; (**B**) focal CNS injury; (**C**) multifocal CNS injury; (**D**) global CNS injury; and the potential patterns of biomarker kinetics. In panel **A**, we appreciate an early and transient increase in the biomaker, in the rest of the panels the biomarker peaks and is detected for longer period of time. CNS: central nervous system, CEA: carotid endarterectomy, CAS: Carotid artery stenting, and CPB: cardiopulmonary bypass.

CNS, but recent evidence indicates that it is also present in the human gut, specifically in enteric glial cells.

S100B has intracellular and extracellular targets and has autocrine and paracrine effects on glia, neurons, and microglia. All physiological actions (neurotrophic effects) appear to be exerted at nanomolar concentrations; in contrast, micromolar concentrations of the protein are found after cell damage. S100 has been considered a marker of generalized blood–brain barrier (BBB) dysfunction because it is present and secreted by astrocytes into the CSF after CNS injury.[4] Increased serum and CSF concentrations are observed after focal or global injury of the CNS, and sustained elevations of S100B have been reported in patients with large brain infarcts. This last phenomenon may be explained by the fact that after severe ischemic infarcts, there is a period of ischemic expansion involving the penumbra area with further release of the protein.[5]

Recent preclinical studies demonstrate that extracerebral ischemia and reperfusion, bone trauma, and sepsis also trigger the release of S100B, which suggests an extracranial origin of S100B or the possibility of BBB dysfunction induced by remote ischemia-reperfusion. Moreover, S100B has been considered an acute-phase reactant as its serum concentrations are increased in response to inflammatory conditions even without structural damage to the CNS. This phenomenon has been illustrated by experiments in humans in whom lipopolysaccharide was administered to mimic endotoxemia, resulting in S100B spikes along with other proinflammatory cytokines.

To make things ever more complicated, there is evidence from studies in rodents anesthetized with thiopental suggesting that the concentrations of S100B in the brain are much higher than in those anesthetized with either halothane or ketamine.[6] In humans, neither sevoflurane nor propofol appear to have an impact on the systemic concentrations of S100B.

The systemic concentrations of S100B are influenced by modifiable and nonmodifiable factors such as genetic susceptibility, age, gender, and chronic hypertension. For instance, the concentrations of S100B are higher in ApoE

4 carriers (a genotype associated with dementia) than in those with ApoE 2 and 3.[7] Perhaps more importantly, worse outcomes are observed in patients carrying the ApoE genotype after neurologic insults. Patients with chronic hypertension and cervical or intracranial artery stenosis may have an exaggerated rise in S100B after mild or no CNS injury due to lack of autoregulation and subsequent predisposition to BBB damage.[8] This phenomenon has also been demonstrated in the setting of cardiac surgery without cardiopulmonary bypass (CPB) in which patients with cerebrovascular atherosclerotic disease show a significantly higher, although, temporary release of S100B than those without cerebrovascular disease.

Finally, the S100B protein can be measured in blood and CSF and has a half-life of 25 minutes. Its elimination is not affected by moderate renal dysfunction.

S100B PROTEIN IN THE PERIOPERATIVE PERIOD OF CARDIAC AND THORACOABDOMINAL AORTIC SURGERY

Postoperative cerebral lesions indicating embolic phenomena can be observed in approximately one third of patients who undergo cardiac surgery, but not all embolic injuries translate into focal neurologic deficits. Moreover, whether microembolic events directly correlate with cognitive deficits is also unknown.

Clinical studies indicate that the cerebral tissue and systemic concentrations of S100B increase during and after cardiac surgery and perhaps even more after long periods of total circulatory arrest.[9] However, there is still debate as to whether the rise in systemic concentrations of S100B represents cerebral insult (global cerebral hypoperfusion or embolic stroke) or release from extracerebral sources as several clinical studies demonstrate that the concentrations of this protein are increased even when circulatory measures to protect the brain are implemented.

High systemic concentrations of S100B have been associated with increased length of stay, morbidity, and mortality. Jonsson et al. found an odds ratio for death and survival of 15.75 when they used 0.5 µg/L as the cutoff value.[10] Results from studies that have looked at S100B as a predictor of neurologic outcomes after cardiac surgery are controversial even though data suggest that this biomarker has a sensitivity and specificity of approximately 90% to predict cerebral lesions and correlates with brain infarct size.

POCD and delirium are common neurologic complications after cardiac surgery. The prognostic and predictive value of S100B as a marker of these complications is poorly understood. A large observational study and two

randomized control trials found no correlation between preoperative or postoperative S100B systemic concentrations and neuropsychological outcomes.[11] This contrasts with data regarding postoperative memory decline, which suggest that an elevated S100B 7 hours post-CPB is an effective predictor of that outcome.[12]

Spinal cord ischemia during thoracoabdominal aortic aneurysm (TAAA) surgery is a feared complication with the potentially devastating consequence of paraplegia. The most commonly used strategy to detect spinal cord ischemia during this procedure is monitoring of motor and sensory evoked potentials, but this methodology is very insensitive despite its high specificity.[13] Thus, several groups of researchers have investigated the kinectics and prognostic and predictive value of S100B in patients undergoing TAAA surgery with or without left atrio-pulmonary vein–femoral artery bypass. Briefly, S100B appears to peak in patients with spinal cord lesions who develop neurologic complications. Unfortunately, the concentrations of this biomarker begin to increase after the onset of clinical symptoms, a finding that again questions the utility of S100B as an early marker for such outcomes.

S100B AND NONCARDIAC SURGERY

The study of neurologic complications after carotid surgery is of interest, even though the incidence of ischemic stroke after carotid endarterectomy is low. Current modalities for the direct or indirect detection of changes in cerebral blood flow and perfusion rely on continuous intraoperative neurologic assessment (in awake patients) or measurement of electrical potentials, regional cerebral oxygen saturation, and blood flow velocities (in anesthetized patients). Unfortunately, some of these techniques cannot always be used because of some patient characteristics, surgeon preference, or lack of knowledge in their use.

The results regarding use of S100B to detect brain ischemia and predict outcomes after carotid endarterectomy (CEA) remain controversial. It has been hypothesized that a transient episode of cerebral hypoperfusion during CEA is associated with BBB dysfunction, which would trigger the early and usually post-clamping release of S100B.[14] But unfortunately the minimum magnitude of the ischemic event needed to open the BBB and induce the subsequent release of S100B it is unknown. Moreover, the correlation of S100B with electroencephalographic changes is poor, hence it is possible that intraoperative or early postoperative spikes of S100B after CEA are multifactorial. What appears clearer is that after carotid artery stenting procedures, the rise in the concentrations of S100B is higher than during

CEA. This may be explained by the fact that in carotid artery stenting the microembolic load is significantly larger, hence the ischemic volume.[14] The S100B protein has also been investigated in the context of subarachnoid hemorrhage (SAH), but this biomarker by itself has failed to predict delayed cerebral ischemia, vasospasm, and functional neurologic outcomes.

The predictive value of S100B in patients undergoing spine surgery for conditions including chronic cervical myelopathy and intra- or extramedullary tumors is not conclusive. More promising results have been found in patients with subacute spinal cord lesions. In this setting, S100B is an acute-phase protein with a double pattern of release (Figure 13.2). One pattern occurs after the acute injury of the spinal cord and is characterized by an initial spike in its concentrations, followed by normalization of its levels only if the treatment initiated to ameliorate the injury is effective. The second pattern is characterized by a sustained postoperative increase (48 hours or longer) of S100B after spinal cord injury; this pattern is observed in cases of sustained damaged to the spinal cord. Supporting the concept of S100B as an acute-phase reactant marker, Saranteas et al. found that serum concentrations of S100B rose postoperatively after extensive oral and maxillofacial reconstruction in fashion similar to that of other acute-phase reactant markers and proinflammatory cytokines such as C-reactive protein, IL-6, and IL-1β.[15]

S100B AND SEPSIS

Sepsis and multiorgan failure are potential complications of major surgeries. Commonly, septic patients show some degree of CNS dysfunction, referred to as sepsis-associated encephalopathy. Thus, several investigators have shown interest in the diagnostic and predictive value of S100B in that setting. Several reports indicate that S100B is increased in patients with sepsis and in volunteers treated with lipopolysaccharide, findings suggesting that S100B reflects, as expected, glial inflammation. However, the release of S100B in the context of sepsis is likely multifactorial, reflecting glial reaction to systemic hypotension (cerebral hypoperfusion) and the action of inflammatory cytokines on the BBB (Figure 13.1).

The ability of S100B to predict clinical outcomes in the context of sepsis is unclear. Data from clinical studies indicate that S100B correlates with low levels of consciousness in septic patients but not with electroencephalographic or Glasgow Coma Score changes.

NEURON-SPECIFIC ENOLASE (NSE)

GENERAL CONCEPTS

NSE is a dimeric enzyme found in neurons and neuroendocrine cells. Only the subunits α and γ of the enzyme are specific for neurons. The molecular weight of NSE is 78 kDa; it can be measured in serum and CSF and its half-life is significantly longer than that of S100B (24 hours). As with S100B, genetic factors may have an impact on the release of NSE in the perioperative period.[16] Age affects the CSF concentrations of this biomarker; there is an increase of 1% per year, which explains why elderly patients have a higher concentration than younger patients. Several researchers have investigated the effect of anesthetic techniques and anesthetics on the release of NSE before and after minor surgery. Remarkably, general anesthesia is associated with higher systemic concentrations of NSE than local anesthesia but, similar to S100B, neither sevoflurane nor propofol appear to affect the release of NSE.[17]

Serum levels of NSE between 2 and 20 μg/L are considered normal, higher than 30 μg/L is pathologic, and 115 μg/L or higher is associated with poor prognosis.[18] NSE is increased in the serum after various neurologic insults, including global cerebral hypoperfusion (cardiac

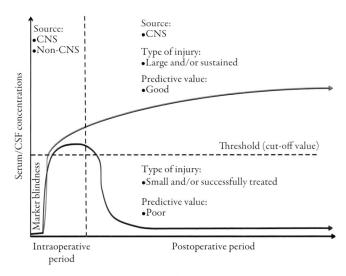

Figure 13.2 This figure depicts two different patterns of marker kinetics. One of the curves represents a biomarker that has an early and transient period of detection, the other curve illustrates a different kinetic that is characterized by an early and sustained period of detection. This last curve would be associated, perhaps, with a better predictive value. The marker blindness period is the time between the CNS insult and the moment that the marker is reliable measured in serum or CSF. Ideally, the blidness period should be short to detect early insults and hence initiate early therapeutic interventios. CSF: Cerebral spinal fluid, CNS: central nervous system.

arrest), repetitive head trauma, temporal lobe epilepsy, and focal injury (ischemic strokes and SAH). Recent practice guidelines indicate that NSE serum levels higher than 33 μg/L are predictive of poor neurologic outcomes after cardiac arrest.[19] Similar results have been reported in patients with ischemic and hemorrhagic strokes in whom elevated concentrations of NSE correlated with poor functional outcomes. In contrast, NSE does not appear to have a predictive value in patients with SAH.

NSE PROTEIN IN THE PERIOPERATIVE PERIOD OF CARDIAC AND TAAA SURGERY

Serum and CSF levels of NSE rise during cardiac surgery with CPB and return to baseline values 24 hours postoperatively. Serum levels of NSE in the context of CPB may have two different sources: neuronal and non-neuronal (or extracerebral). Red blood cells and platelets are a source of NSE; thus hemolysis during CPB and the use of cardiotomy suction may result in the release of NSE. As expected, off-pump cardiac surgery is often associated with significantly lower levels of NSE. Also, the release of NSE during CPB may reflect the inflammatory state associated with this technique. This suggests that NSE may, as with S100B, act as an acute-phase reactant mainly when the perioperative pattern of release is temporary. Supporting this concept are results obtained from a randomized, controlled trial in which patients underwent preoperative exposure to hyperbaric oxygen or no exposure. Those assigned to the hyperbaric oxygen regimen showed significantly lower serum concentrations of NSE than those in controls. The reinfusion of processed cell-saver blood may be responsible for a substantial increase in the serum concentrations of NSE, since recovered blood from the surgical field contains elevated levels of proinflammatory factors. The release of NSE is also affected by body temperature. It is unknown whether this is the result of hypothermia itself or the fact that patients undergoing deep hypothermic CPB undergo larger surgical procedures with longer pump runs or have a higher risk of cerebral ischemia.

Several investigators have assessed the predictive value of NSE following cardiac surgery, and the results are controversial. Remarkably, in most of the studies, the average maximum postoperative concentrations of NSE are within "normal" limits, suggesting that "significant damage" to the CNS has not occurred intraoperatively to trigger the release of the enzyme. Only a small proportion of patients has shown serum concentrations of 30 μg/L or higher. Even in highly embolic interventions such as

transfemoral aortic valve placement, the average peak of NSE remains within normal limits. This finding suggests again that the total volume of ischemia is not high enough to trigger significant release of NSE or, less likely, that recovery occurs without significant progression of the infarcts. Of note, most patients remain asymptomatic, which indicates that most emboli occur in noneloquent areas of the brain.

The predictive value of NSE has also been investigated in aortic aneurysm surgical repair, but, as occurs with S100B, NSE does not appear to add information beyond that obtained by transcranial motor-evoked potentials monitoring. Moreover, the concentrations of NSE in the CSF of patients undergoing descending thoracic or thoracoabdominal aorta repair are increased independent of the neurologic symptoms.

Several investigators have measured the systemic concentrations of NSE in patients undergoing implantable cardiac defibrillator implantation in an attempt to assess whether temporary periods of cardiac arrest trigger the release of NSE and if that correlates with neurologic outcomes. Remarkably, the increase in NSE was associated with the number of shocks and the cumulative time in circulatory arrest and cognitive dysfunction.

NSE IN THE CONTEXT OF NONCARDIAC SURGERY

Most studies have shown that 1) higher preoperative NSE concentrations are observed in patients with a higher degree of carotid stenosis; 2) the enzyme increases after surgery; 3) as with S100B, significantly higher concentrations are found after carotid artery stenting, although this last finding is controversial; and 4) the predictive value of NSE after carotid surgery is unclear.[14] It is important to note that the postoperative peak levels of NSE are also higher in patients undergoing CEA under general anesthesia than in those undergoing local anesthesia, which suggests a potential effect of anesthetics on the release of the enzyme. However, this interpretation is purely speculative.[17]

The role of NSE in predicting neurologic outcomes in noncardiac nonvascular surgery is also poorly understood. Studies suggest that after minor or noncomplicated surgery, serum or CSF concentrations of NSE concentrations remain unchanged even in patients who develop POCD. In contrast, in larger and more invasive interventions such as orthotopic liver transplantation, NSE levels correlate well with low regional cerebral oxygen saturations. However, it is unknown whether NSE can predict neurologic outcomes after this type of surgery.

NSE has also been the focus of investigations of sepsis and septic shock. Preclinical and clinical data indicate that the enzyme peaks during sepsis but, unfortunately, there is very little or no clinically relevant information regarding the predictive value of the enzyme in relation to clinical outcomes.

TAU PROTEIN

GENERAL CONCEPTS

Tau is a microtubule-associated protein that acts as a stabilizer of axonal microtubules. Tau has multiple isoforms, and its phosphorylation occurs in association with neuronal death. The kinetics appear to be different from those of NSE and S100B; these last two usually show an early (within 24 hours) peak after CNS injury, whereas Tau can only be detected 48 hours or longer after injury. Tau elevations are observed in neurodegenerative disorders such as Alzheimer's disease and in non-neurodegenerative disorders.[20]

The predictive value of Tau protein has been demonstrated in patients with traumatic brain injury in whom a microdialysis catheter was inserted into the brain tissue. In this type of neurologic insult, the Tau protein showed low (70%) sensitivity but high (100%) specificity for predicting poor clinical outcomes. A similar sensitivity and specificity has been found in the prediction of poor neurologic outcomes after cardiac arrest. In contrast to the observations in traumatic brain injury and cardiac arrest, Tau has a poor predictive value after stroke. Anesthetics may promote abnormal hyperphosphorylation of Tau, although these data were obtained with older anesthetics such as ether and pentobarbital.

TAU AND CARDIAC SURGERY

Tau protein increases during the perioperative period of cardiac surgery;[21] its levels peak in the postoperative period and return to baseline by the fourth postoperative day. Importantly, serum levels of Tau are higher in patients with postoperative cognitive disorders.[21]

Tau levels have also been investigated in patients undergoing aortic surgery. Shiiya et al. demonstrated that elevations of CSF Tau protein after thoracic or thoracoabdominal aortic surgery were higher in those with brain infarction than in neurologically intact patients. They also found statistically significant differences between the patients with transient neurologic deficits and those without deficits.[22]

TAU, NONCARDIAC SURGERY, AND SPESIS

No studies have assessed the kinetics and predictive value of Tau protein in the context of noncardiac surgery. Only preclinical information indicates that surgery may trigger phosphorylation of Tau in the hippocampus. This finding suggests that this change may participate in postoperative cognitive decline.

METALLOPROTEINASES (MMPS)

GENERAL CONCEPTS

Metalloproteinases (MMPs) are zinc-dependent endopeptidases secreted by various cells, including myocytes, endothelial cells, and macrophages.[23] The MMPs are divided into subgroups: gelatinases (MMP-2, -9), collagenases (MMP-1, -8, -13), matrilysins (MMP-7), membrane-type MMPs (MMP-14, -15, -16, -17), and others (MMP-11, -12).

Serum levels of MMP-9 peak early in patients with stroke, and they strongly correlate with neuronal death in areas of secondary injury. MMP-9 is also increased after traumatic brain injury and SAH; remarkably, neurologic outcomes are better after enzyme levels in the brain are reduced after administration of anti-inflammatory agents. Interestingly, sevoflurane preconditioning has been associated with reduction in MMP-9 levels in the brain and improvement in BBB permeability, suggesting that MMP-9 is a marker of BBB dysfunction. Surgical stress and proinflammatory factors, including IL-1β, IL-8 and TNF-α, stimulate the release and enzymatic activity of MMP-9.[24]

MMP-9 AND CARDIAC SURGERY

Little is known about the predictive implications of MMP-9 on clinical outcomes. Circulating concentrations of MMP-9 spike immediately after CPB, perhaps as a consequence of the contact of leukocytes with the extracorporeal circuit; thus the enzyme may be used as a marker of systemic inflammatory response. Higher circulating concentrations of the enzyme are observed in patients who develop postoperative neuropsychological disorders.

MMP-9 AND NONCARDIAC SURGERY

The expression of MMP-9 mRNA in leukocytes is also increased after nonvascular surgery, perhaps as an indication of the perioperative inflammatory response. Interestingly, women undergoing breast surgery under propofol-paravertebral block anesthesia show a lower circulating concentration of the enzyme than those receiving sevoflurane-opioid anesthesia. This finding suggests that an anesthesia technique with anti-inflammatory effects can modulate the release of MMP-9.

The serum levels of MMP-9 peak during CEA and correlate with duration of carotid occlusion.[25] A prospective cohort study showed that patients with cognitive dysfunction after carotid surgery had higher preoperative and postoperative plasma levels of MMP-9 than in those without cognitive symptoms. In the setting of CEA, postoperative increments of MMP-9 can represent 1) systemic inflammatory response, 2) local release of the protein due to atherosclerotic plaque manipulation, and 3) microembolization or transient ischemia leading to BBB dysfunction. However, the finding of higher preoperative levels in patients who developed POCD may represent a higher "baseline" inflammatory state or silent areas of ischemia associated with subclinical BBB dysfunction. This is supported by work from Taurino et al., who found that asymptomatic patients with higher preoperative levels of MMP-9 had significantly more cerebral lesions than those without such levels.[26]

MMP-9 AND SEPSIS

Not surprisingly, local and systemic concentrations of MMP-9 are increased during sepsis. Proinflammatory cytokines such as TNF-α have been shown to increase the cerebral expression of MMP-9, which in turn increases the permeability of the BBB. In a model of encephalopathy, MMP-9 played a significant role in the development of cognitive deficits.

Unfortunately, there is no information regarding the predictive value of MMP-9 for short- and long-term neurologic outcomes associated with sepsis.

UBIQUITIN C TERMINAL HYDROXYLASE-L1 (UCH-L1)

UCH-L1 is a highly specific neuronal protein that functions as an enzyme.[27] An extraneuronal form of the enzyme can be found in small quantities in the testes. The enzyme can be measured in serum and CSF as early as 6 hours after the neurologic insult and for approximately 7 days thereafter. For instance, levels of the enzyme increase through the second week after SAH and beyond.[28] In stroke patients, the enzyme performed better than S100B in terms of reflecting response to treatment and correlating with clinical outcomes. In patients with traumatic brain injury, UCH-L1 has shown correlation with severity of the disease and survival.

To date, there are no studies assessing either the predictive value of UCH-L1 in the perioperative period or the effect of anesthetics on UCH-L1 biology and kinetics.

FUTURE DIRECTIONS: A PANEL OF NEURONAL BIOMARKERS?

As presented in previous sections, the use of a single biomarker to predict short- and long-term neurologic outcomes is associated with poor sensitivity and relatively high specificity. Factors including differences in cellular, and subcellular localizations of each biomarker in different areas of the CNS may explain in part the low predictive ability of single markers. Moreover, there is a period after neuronal injury when single markers may not be identified (marker blindness) (Figure 13.2). For instance, most of the biomarkers studied may peak several hours after the insult, thus delaying diagnosis and treatment. A panel of neurobiomarkers expressed in neurons and/or glial cells would be an alternative for improving the predictive ability (area under the receiver operating characteristic curve) and could provide information regarding potential localization of areas of CNS insult. Further research here is warranted.

A recent study demonstrated that a panel of six biomarkers predicted cerebral vasospasm, infarction, and poor functional outcomes after SAH.[29] The panel included the neuronal proteins 14-3-3β, 14-3ζ, CCSntf, CCSctf, NSE, and UCH-L1. In the perioperative setting, a panel of biomarkers has also shown promising results. In the vast majority of patients undergoing aortic surgery under CPB with deep hypothermic cardiac arrest, 14-3-3β, 14-3ζ, pNFH (hypophosphorylated form of the high-molecular-weight neurofilament subunit), and UCH-L1 are increased in the CSF. In those undergoing CPB without cardiac arrest but having neurologic complications, the same biomarkers show a rise in their CSF concentrations; in those patients with neurologic complications the rise in all biomarkers precedes the onset of clinical symptoms.

CONCLUSIONS

Physicians and researchers involved in the perioperative care of patients have encountered two major obstacles in the attempt to predict postoperative neurologic outcomes in patients at risk of neurologic insults. First, we have not been able to quantify CNS reserve in the preoperative period. Second, we have struggled to measure or quantify damage based on detection of neurobiomarkers. Moreover, transient episodes of ischemia or mild neurotoxic injury may be associated with "leakage" of biomarkers primarily into the CSF and, less likely, into serum. In these cases of biomarker "leakage," the patient may recover after the insult, which suggests reversible neuronal damage (Figure 13.1A).

More than eight different neurologic biomarkers have been studied in the perioperative period. Unfortunately, the investigations on S100B, NSE, and Tau protein have shown mixed results. There are several reasons that could explain the conflicting findings. First, individual differences based on genetic polymorphisms may explain why some patients show elevations of a specific marker compared to that in other patients. Second, potential sources of "contamination" such as non-neural S100B may confound the laboratory findings. Third, different assays may have different sensitivities to detect levels of S100B, NSE, Tau, and UCH-L1 protein. Thus, the results reported by different authors may not be comparable. Perhaps the use of a panel of biomarkers will help overcome the limitations of using a single neurobiomarker until the CNS "troponin" is found in the future. More research is warranted to identify and validate the use of these markers.

CONFLICT OF INTEREST STATEMENT

J.C. has no conflicts of interest to disclose.

REFERENCES

1. Cata JP, Abdelmalak B, Farag E. Neurological biomarkers in the perioperative period. *Br J Anaesth.* 2008;107(6):844–858.
2. DeCaprio AP. Biomarkers: coming of age for environmental health and risk assessment. *Environ Sci Technol.* 1997;31(7):1837–1848.
3. Moore BW. A soluble protein characteristic of the nervous system. *Biochem Biophys Res Commun.* 2008;19(6):739–744.
4. Kapural M, Krizanac-Bengez L, Barnett G, et al. Serum S-100beta as a possible marker of blood-brain barrier disruption. *Brain Res.* 2008;940(1-2):102–104.
5. Fassbender K, Schmidt R, Schreiner A, et al. Leakage of brain-originated proteins in peripheral blood: temporal profile and diagnostic value in early ischemic stroke. *J Neurol Sci.* 2008;148(1):101–105.
6. Vicente E, Tramontina F, Leite MC, et al. S100B levels in the cerebrospinal fluid of rats are sex and anaesthetic dependent. *Clin Exp Pharmacol Physiol.* 2008;34(11):1126–1130.
7. Kofke WA, Konitzer P, Meng QC, Guo J, Cheung A. The effect of apolipoprotein E genotype on neuron specific enolase and S-100beta levels after cardiac surgery. *Anesth Analg.* 2008;99(5):1323–1325; table of contents.
8. Schmidt M, Scheunert T, Steinbach G, et al. Hypertension as a risk factor for cerebral injury during cardiopulmonary bypass. Protein S100B and transcranial Doppler findings. *Anaesthesia.* 2008;56(8):733–738.
9. Bhattacharya K, Westaby S, Pillai R, Standing SJ, Johnsson P, Taggart DP. Serum S100B and hypothermic circulatory arrest in adults. *Ann Thorac Surg.* 2008;68(4):1225–1229.
10. Jonsson H, Johnsson P, Birch-Iensen M, Alling C, Westaby S, Blomquist S. S100B as a predictor of size and outcome of stroke after cardiac surgery. *Ann Thorac Surg.* 2008;71(5):1433–1437.
11. Carrier M, Denault A, Lavoie J, Perrault LP. Randomized controlled trial of pericardial blood processing with a cell-saving device on neurologic markers in elderly patients undergoing coronary artery bypass graft surgery. *Ann Thorac Surg.* 2008;82(1):51–55.
12. Svenmarker S, Sandstrom E, Karlsson T, Aberg T. Is there an association between release of protein S100B during cardiopulmonary bypass and memory disturbances? *Scand Cardiovasc J.* 2008;36(2):117–122.
13. Keyhani K, Miller CC, 3rd, Estrera AL, Wegryn T, Sheinbaum R, Safi HJ. Analysis of motor and somatosensory evoked potentials during thoracic and thoracoabdominal aortic aneurysm repair. *J Vasc Surg.* 2008;49(1):36–41.
14. Brightwell RE, Sherwood RA, Athanasiou T, Hamady M, Cheshire NJ. The neurological morbidity of carotid revascularisation: using markers of cellular brain injury to compare CEA and CAS. *Eur J Vasc Endovasc Surg.* 2008;34(5):552–560.
15. Saranteas T, Tachmintzis A, Katsikeris N, et al. Perioperative thyroid hormone kinetics in patients undergoing major oral and maxillofacial operations. *J Oral Maxillofac Surg.* 2008;65(3):408–414.
16. McDonagh DL, Mathew JP, White WD, et al. Cognitive function after major noncardiac surgery, apolipoprotein E4 genotype, and biomarkers of brain injury. *Anesthesiology.* 2008;112(4):852–859.
17. Wijeyaratne SM, Collins MA, Barth JH, Gough MJ. Jugular venous neurone specific enolase (NSE) increases following carotid endarterectomy under general, but not local, anaesthesia. *Eur J Vasc Endovasc Surg.* 2008;38(3):262–266.
18. Schaarschmidt H, Prange HW, Reiber H. Neuron-specific enolase concentrations in blood as a prognostic parameter in cerebrovascular diseases. *Stroke.* 2008;25(3):558–565.
19. Wijdicks EF, Hijdra A, Young GB, Bassetti CL, Wiebe S. Practice parameter: prediction of outcome in comatose survivors after cardiopulmonary resuscitation (an evidence-based review): report of the Quality Standards Subcommittee of the American Academy of Neurology. *Neurology.* 2008;67(2):203–210.
20. Planel E, Richter KE, Nolan CE, et al. Anesthesia leads to tau hyperphosphorylation through inhibition of phosphatase activity by hypothermia. *J Neurosci.* 2008;27(12):3090–3097.
21. Ramlawi B, Rudolph JL, Mieno S, et al. Serologic markers of brain injury and cognitive function after cardiopulmonary bypass. *Ann Surg.* 2008;244(4):593–601.
22. Shiiya N, Kunihara T, Miyatake T, Matsuzaki K, Yasuda K. Tau protein in the cerebrospinal fluid is a marker of brain injury after aortic surgery. *Ann Thorac Surg.* 2008;77(6):2034–2038.
23. Goetzl EJ, Banda MJ, Leppert D. Matrix metalloproteinases in immunity. *J Immunol.* 2008;156(1):1–4.
24. Sasajima K, Futami R, Matsutani T, et al. Increases in soluble tumor necrosis factor receptors coincide with increases in interleukin-6 and proteinases after major surgery. *Hepatogastroenterology.* 2008;56(94–95):1377–1381.
25. Ishigaki D, Ogasawara K, Suga Y, et al. Concentration of matrix metalloproteinase-9 in the jugular bulb during carotid endarterectomy correlates with severity of intraoperative cerebral ischemia. *Cerebrovasc Dis.* 2008;25(6):587–592.
26. Taurino M, Raffa S, Mastroddi M, et al. Metalloproteinase expression in carotid plaque and its correlation with plasma levels before and after carotid endarterectomy. *Vasc Endovascular Surg.* 2008;41(6):516–521.
27. Thompson RJ, Doran JF, Jackson P, Dhillon AP, Rode J. PGP 9.5—a new marker for vertebrate neurons and neuroendocrine cells. *Brain Res.* 2008;278(1-2):224–228.
28. Lewis SB, Wolper R, Chi YY, et al. Identification and preliminary characterization of ubiquitin C terminal hydrolase 1 (UCHL1) as a biomarker of neuronal loss in aneurysmal subarachnoid hemorrhage. *J Neurosci Res.* 2008;88(7):1475–1484.
29. Siman R, Giovannone N, Toraskar N, et al. Evidence that a panel of neurodegeneration biomarkers predicts vasospasm, infarction, and outcome in aneurysmal subarachnoid hemorrhage. *PLoS One.* 2008;6(12):e28938.

INDEX